How to S
in Medicin

Personally and professionally

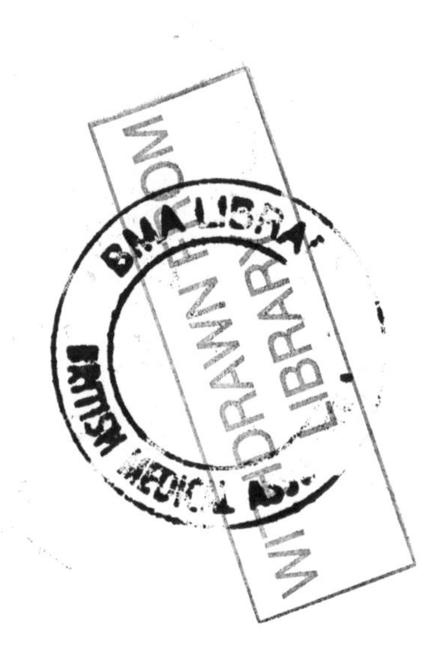

Professor Jenny Firth-Cozens is an occupational and clinical psychologist who has worked throughout the health service and within academia. In addition to a number of studies of MRC funded interventions for occupational stress and depression, she conducted and reported the first UK study of stress in young doctors, following them for almost 20 years and providing an understanding of the problems that face doctors throughout their careers. She has been special advisor and consultant to London Deanery, the National Clinical Assessment Service and the National Patient Safety Agency. She has published numerous scientific articles and reports along with several books, both academic and popular, including *Stress in Health Professionals: Psychological and Organizational Causes and Interventions* (Wiley) *and Nervous Breakdown: What Is It? What Causes It? Who Will Help?* (Piatkus) which was a book club choice for many years. In addition she has contributed articles and columns to most leading newspapers and magazines.

Dr. Jamie Harrison is a GP and Deputy Director of Postgraduate GP Education for the Northern Deanery. He pioneered the GP Career Start Scheme in County Durham and for five years advised the English Department of Health on GP recruitment in Europe. He has collaborated extensively to produce a range of books on contemporary health service issues, publishing *Medical Vocation and Generation X, GP Tomorrow, Clinical Governance in Primary Care, The New GP, and Rebuilding Trust in Healthcare.* He continues to work closely with young doctors as a GP Trainer, as well as supporting older doctors with performance concerns.

How to Survive in Medicine

Personally and professionally

Jenny Firth-Cozens, MSc, PhD, FBPsS
Special Advisor on Postgraduate Medical Education
London Deanery of Postgraduate Medical and Dental Education
London, UK

With

Jamie Harrison MA FRCGP
Deputy Director of Postgraduate GP Education
The Northern Deanery
Newcastle upon Tyne, UK

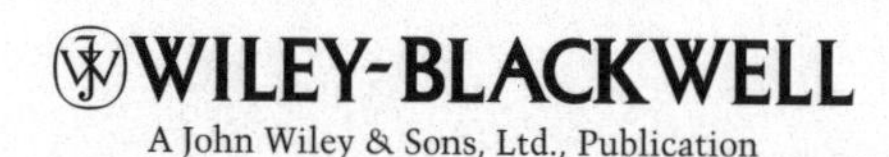

BMJ | Books

BMJ Books is an imprint of BMJ Publishing Group Limited, used under licence by Blackwell Publishing which was acquired by John Wiley & Sons in February 2007. Blackwell's publishing programme has been merged with Wiley's global Scientific, Technical and Medical business to form Wiley-Blackwell.

Registered office: John Wiley & Sons Ltd, The Atrium, Southern Gate, Chichester, West Sussex, PO19 8SQ, UK

Editorial offices: 9600 Garsington Road, Oxford, OX4 2DQ, UK
111 River Street, Hoboken, NJ 07030-5774, USA
The Atrium, Southern Gate, Chichester, West Sussex, PO19 8SQ, UK

For details of our global editorial offices, for customer services and for information about how to apply for permission to reuse the copyright material in this book please see our website at www.wiley.com/wiley-blackwell

Library of Congress Cataloging-in-Publication Data

Firth-Cozens, Jenny.
How to survive in medicine : personally and professionally / Jenny Firth-Cozens ; with contributions from Jamie Harrison.
p. ; cm.
Includes bibliographical references and index.
ISBN 978-1-4051-9271-2
1. Physicians—Vocational guidance. 2. Physicians—Job stress. I. Title.
[DNLM: 1. Physicians—psychology. 2. Interprofessional Relations. 3. Stress, Psychological—prevention & control. W 62 F527h 2010]
R690.F566 2010
610.69023—dc22

2010000504

ISBN: 978-1-4051-9271-2

A catalogue record for this book is available from the British Library.

Set in 9.5/12pt Minion by MPS Limited, A Macmillan Company

Printed and bound in Malaysia by Vivar Printing Sdn Bhd
1 2010

Contents

Introduction

In the early 1980s I was working for the Medical Research Council at Sheffield University, looking at psychotherapy interventions for work-based depression. Two doctors in specialty training at the local hospital came to see me to ask if anything could be done about their profession: something, they said, was wrong. Over the past two months two young doctors they knew had killed themselves. Despite the shattering effects they felt about this, nothing had been said in their teams; they just met and talked clinically as usual. Both incidents were treated as if nothing had happened; as if doctors were uniformly strong and so couldn't possibly be depressed or take their own lives. Nor, it seemed, should they be stressed by the loss of a colleague. They asked if I could start a study which tested this presumption, that explored the causes of stress and depression in doctors, and investigated what could be done about it.

My research interest at the time was to see which causes of stress and depression were job-related and which ones the individual brought with them – was it the person, or was it the job? – and so I began a 17 year longitudinal study, following over 300 doctors from their fourth year in medical school to senior doctor posts. Many of the findings in this book, and most of the quotes, come from this study and from the many others which followed.

So, is there a problem?

Medicine is a career that most people consider to be enviable. Whatever one's criteria for a good job, being a doctor ticks a lot of boxes: doctors are needed, respected, well remunerated and can make a difference between life and death. When asked what they enjoyed most about their roles, young doctors said that feeling useful and tackling problems were the most satisfying: 'Finishing a job and knowing that I've done it well'. Many of them also said how much they enjoyed the patients: 'Meeting a lot of people and helping them'. This changes over their careers so that patients and their relatives are often seen as the problem, rather than the benefit of the job. Still, the main enjoyment they experienced should go on: throughout your career you can get satisfaction from being useful and doing things well.

Older doctors when asked the same question often reflected on their role as privileged: 'Where else could I get such variety – every patient's different. It's always interesting, always a challenge.' Others welcomed the detective work involved in diagnosis. General practitioners appreciated the relationships that were formed: 'Caring for three generations of one family' and 'Being able to journey with people through the good times and the bad'. While some felt the increasing pressure from the health care system created real issues for them, others still relished the challenge of beating the system: 'Keeping the needs of the patients ahead of the forces of management'.

It seems then that there are many real satisfactions in medicine which, it might be thought, would outweigh most of the difficulties that you may have to face in your career. A proportion of doctors would agree with this and say that they are 'happy' or 'very happy' with their choice of career: a BMJ survey in 2001 found that 16% of doctors in the United Kingdom, 4% in Spain, 34% in Ireland and 36% in New Zealand were in this satisfied group. However, that is hardly a resounding gold star for great career satisfaction and, at the other extreme, two thirds of British doctors and more than half in many other countries reported feeling unhappy or very unhappy.

There is clearly something about the work or the people who do it, or both, that makes this potentially rewarding career less of a pleasure and satisfaction than you or the rest of the population might expect. This book explores what the pitfalls and problems of medicine are, and how you, the individual doctor, can tackle them. At the very least this should help you to survive your career as a reasonably healthy person; at best it should help you to gain even greater satisfaction and enjoyment from it.

Long-term studies show that dissatisfaction and general unhappiness are, without interventions, remarkably consistent over a lifetime. Although they are not clinical conditions, they do incorporate other more serious problems such as high levels of stress and depression. In numerous surveys around the world doctors who, with their income and educational levels, should be one of the least stressed groups, have levels of stress considerably higher than those of workers in general. Surveys have been remarkably consistent in showing that around 28% of doctors at various points in their careers are above threshold on the General Health Questionnaire (the GHQ is a brief assessment tool which is a useful measure of occupational stress and a snapshot of general psychological problems in a population) compared with 18% for the British workforce as a whole.

Stress is an overused word, but still a useful one as it represents the whole gamut of emotional distress. When it's used in this book it doesn't refer to feelings of pressure or challenge, both of which are inevitable and often positive responses to difficult aspects of life. When stress is mentioned, it's always regarded as negative. Of those who score above threshold on the GHQ, some will show clinical levels of depression or anxiety.

Different surveys of depression in doctors have used very different measures and so it's difficult to be accurate about the levels found. Nevertheless, one study of health care staff as a whole reported that, of those above threshold on the GHQ, half had clinical depression or anxiety at interview[1], so the number of doctors suffering in this way at any one time is likely to be considerable. Most surveys show that the proportion of doctors who are depressed is as great as or more than that of the general population, and this is despite the fact that psychological difficulties as a whole reduce as you rise up the social and occupational ladder. When you consider that, with depression, decision-making, concentration and memory are all going to be impaired, this is going to make a doctor's work even more difficult as well as having a knock-on effect for patient care. Moreover, some groups of doctors are particularly high users of alcohol and other drugs and for those who fall into this category, a smooth ride through their careers becomes somewhat less likely. Overall, it has been estimated that, at some point in their careers, around 15% of doctors will be impaired from depression or substance misuse.

Because of policy changes or new training systems, the most stressed or depressed grades vary according to where the pressure lies in different decades. So in the 1980s in particular, the most distressed were in their first postgraduate year when working hours were formidable, while in the last decade stress levels have evened out across grades, though somewhat higher in consultants. New systems of career progression might change this once more. What this means for you is that there is no particular level in medicine where you can sit back and relax; it means that throughout your careers you need to be aware and to care for your own psychological health, not just that of your patients.

About this book

The chapters which follow come from what is now a very large research literature that considers the difficulties and stressors of medicine as a career, but also from studies that look at what interventions are successful in the workplace. They also reflect my experience and finally from my experience as a clinician and coach working with doctors of all ages and other professionals, and Jamie Harrison's work as a partner in general practice and within a postgraduate deanery. The first part sets out the possible causes of problems, and the second part, much larger, goes into various solutions. The bibliographies which follow each chapter contain key references, while the chapters referred to cover most of the others. We hope the book helps you not only to survive medicine, but also to enjoy it more.

Jenny Firth-Cozens
London

[1]Weinberg A, Creed F. Stress and psychiatric disorder in healthcare professionals and hospital staff. *Lancet* 2000;**355**:533–7.

Part 1 **The job and you**

Chapter 1 **It's just a difficult job**

When people become stressed or depressed while doing difficult jobs like medicine, they tend to look around the workplace at others who are doing jobs that seem equally hard but appear to be functioning well, and wonder if their difficulties are simply because of the way they are rather than the work they do. They ask: 'Is it me or is it the job?' This chapter outlines the parts of the job that have been found to cause problems. There's no doubt that many aspects of the roles within medicine are very difficult and often upsetting, and it takes an unusual person not to feel stressed at times.

1.1 Health organisations can be a health hazard

There is good evidence that the organisation you work in can make a difference to how much stress you experience: some medical schools, some specialties and some organisations are less stressful than others. For example, a medical school that formed its students into small consistent groups throughout their clinical years showed far fewer stressed students than one which sent students through in groups of over 40. Similarly, one hospital will cause problems to a much greater proportion of its staff than will another: one study comparing hospital staff in a number of organisations found those above threshold for stress on the General Health Questionnaire (GHQ) varied from 17% to 34% depending on the hospital, whilst a study of newly qualified house officers in London's hospitals found mean GHQ levels varied from 8.1 to 15.3 and this was not to do with hospital size or whether it is modern or old. It seems the management of a hospital has an effect.

Teaching hospitals tend to be more difficult places to work than non-teaching, probably because the competition is so much fiercer between colleagues, and the patients are more ill. But also it is clear from these data that there are going to be management issues which make one hospital a good place, with satisfied staff and low turnover, while another has disgruntled and stressed staff, where rumours and insecurity abound, and relationships are difficult. In all organisations, from banks to hospitals or general practices, these effects are passed down the hierarchy and on to customers or patients – and bounce back in the costs of absence, turnover, mistakes, litigation and complaints. Whether you are student, staff or patient, management clearly matters.

1.2 Life in the team

This is equally true at the team level. You will probably recognise that some teams you have worked in have been good places to be, while others have a number of people off sick, experience frequent back-biting and scapegoating, and rarely deal with conflicts openly or fairly. So what are the criteria for a good team? Studies have found that in a good team:

- Its task is defined and its objectives clear.
- There is participation in decision-making by all members, good communication and frequent interaction between them.
- It meets regularly to review its objectives, methods and effectiveness.
- There is a shared commitment to excellence of patient care.
- Its members trust each other and feel safe to speak their minds.
- It has reasonably clear boundaries and is not too large (ideally fewer than 10 people).
- Its members know who leads it and the leadership is good.
- Its meetings are well conducted.

What a pleasure it is to be in one of those teams: you can work harder, be more innovative and be carried during those times when life events might make you less productive. Group processes are powerful influences on individual actions, equally strong for those teams where the criteria are not met. For example, studies have shown:

- General practitioners (GPs) in poor teams are more likely to opt for early retirement.
- The quality of teamwork is the principal influence on whether junior doctors take sick leave.
- The team can compensate for an individual member's errors over time, so a well-established team is likely to make fewer errors overall, and to identify and deal with the underlying causes.

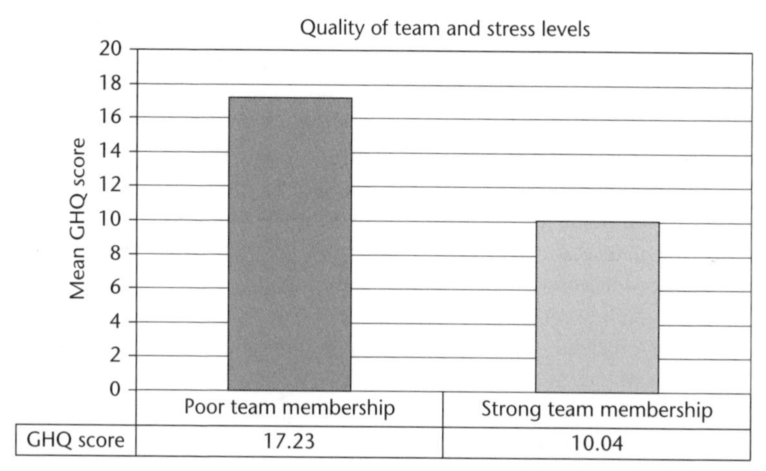

Figure 1.1 GHQ-12 scores for those in good teams compared to poor teams.

- Those in high-quality health care teams are significantly less stressed than those in ineffectively functioning teams or those not in a team – and low stress is related to better patient care.

Some researchers on teams have concluded that, despite all the measures of team function, you really need only to measure the stress levels of its members. Just look at the difference between the stress levels of good teams and poor teams measured on the criteria listed above (Figure 1.1).

Although most health service staff see themselves working in teams, data from the NHS National Staff Surveys show that a large proportion of them work in 'pseudo-teams'; that is, the staff say they are in a team, but it does not meet the criteria for a real team set out above. The surveys show that the fewer criteria that are met, the more those team members make errors and suffer harassment and violence, and the more their organisations show lower quality of care, worse use of resources and higher patient mortality. There are similar findings in primary care. The shift from uni-professional hospital teams, such as a medical firm or a nursing team, to multi-professional groups working within a clinical area to provide a service demands new, more complex teamwork skills which most organisations have not yet managed to develop. So team factors and organisational factors can affect your mental health and always need to be considered.

1.3 Workers of the world

In addition to the sort of organisational and team factors that affect how you feel, there are a number of aspects of a career in medicine which are as stressful as they are in other walks of life. For example, in surveys from most of the western world, **overload** is always said to be difficult – for students, doctors and every other type of staff, whether in health care or outside it. For doctors, the demands are exacerbated by shift work and, when they are young, by frequent relocations. For them the greatest effect of overload is the conflict it can cause between work and home. You probably need more support from home life at a time like this, but you're probably going to get much less than you need because you spend less time at home. This isn't just a factor for women with children: both male and female doctors report equal work–home conflicts.

But even overload – having too few staff and too little time to do the job – doesn't always cause stress; the correlation between hours of work and stress are consistently fairly low in medicine. A young doctor who feels well supported by his or her seniors, who has reasonable periods of sleep, and who gets on with the rest of the staff will usually have no problems working reasonably long hours; in fact, he or she will often really enjoy the feeling of competence growing, of being useful and feeling part of a team. For many people, overload is simply an easy and obvious way to label other less tangible causes, and it's true that it will often play an indirect role in stress in that feeling exhausted will always make other problems loom larger, a death become more distressing. As we shall describe later (Chapter 10), there are many factors that lead an individual to feel overloaded but these rarely include simply the number of hours worked.

Other aspects of your role which cause stress in most types of jobs and most organisations include a **lack of clarity** about what is expected of you – so you don't always know when you've done a good job – and a **lack of discretion or control** in how you carry out that job. The reductions in medical autonomy and increases in accountability that have taken place over the last few decades have made many doctors feel that they no longer have control over their work. A greater sense of personal control leads to increased job satisfaction and even better health. The clearer you are about your role and its expected outcome, the happier you are likely to be; and most of us would rather achieve that outcome in the way that suits us best.

Sexism, racism and homophobia exist in all walks of life and medicine is certainly not immune from them. While this might be more subtle when directed towards sexuality or ethnicity, it can still be remarkably open in terms of women. For example, two female first-year postgraduates wrote:

> *My consultant told me that women are unable to make decisions about male patients, especially if they are life and death decisions. He thought they should stick to paediatrics and dermatology.*

My consultant would put his arm round my waist and pull me to him laughing and saying 'how about a hot date', even though other people were around. I found it really embarrassing and didn't know how to handle it. I didn't want to look like a prude but I knew he shouldn't do it.

1.4 And then there's medicine itself

Beyond these stressors common to workers everywhere are others that are particular to medicine, and some of these vary to some extent depending on where you are in your career. However, the following are always difficult for almost everyone at times.

- **Dealing with difficult patients.** Even before people could look up their symptoms on the Internet, it was still difficult to have to deal with patients or patients' relatives who were argumentative, unappreciative, untrusting or just plain abusive.

Sometime I feel overwhelmed with the total lack of appreciation and even resentment I get from patients. This has got so much worse over the last 20 years as psychiatrists now only get the most psychotic of patients and often have to section people. I guess sometimes the relatives are relieved. (Psychiatrist)

Then there's the 'heartsink' patient with chronic back pain. You just dread them coming back. You know that whatever medication you suggest won't work, and the demand for yet another specialist referral will lead to the same negative outcome. And you get the blame (again) for not sorting it all out. (GP)

As people increasingly consult the Internet before they talk to you, or come in to see you holding a newspaper cutting about the latest treatment or cure, expectations of what you can provide seem to go up and up. Television programmes such as Casualty or ER don't help as they offer false hopes of miraculous medical interventions. The health care scandals of the last decade have made some people less accepting of your opinion, although the general loss of deference in the population towards authority figures may be more at play here. Generally doctors are still one of the most trusted professions by societies across the world.

- **Death and suffering.** If you ask young doctors to complete a questionnaire and rate a number of known stressors, including dealing with death and suffering, they rate this item very low – 'not a problem to me'. But if you ask them to write about a recent stressful event, young doctors in particular write most often about this area, especially if the patient was young or in other ways similar to them. For example:

> *A patient with carcinoma of pancreas, otherwise fit, aged 43, developed a massive coagulopathy after total pancreatectomy. He died. I had feelings of total helplessness while giving blood, etc, although management decisions were not left to me. Could not accept defeat and couldn't cope with total failure of our therapies, despite realising medically the gravity of the situation.*

> *A 29 year old woman, recently married, was presumed to have sarcoidosis, but biopsy showed adenocarcinoma with lung metastases. The consultant reckoned she had six weeks to live. The fact that she was young and female made the incident particularly distressing to come to terms with. Also she was just married and had a devoted husband.*

Of course it's upsetting to see someone die at a time when they shouldn't, or to be in pain or distress from something you have done to them, however necessary it was. It is also difficult on those thankfully rare occasions when someone close to you is ill and the boundary between your personal and professional life becomes blurred. For example, a fourth year medical student wrote:

> *Mother was admitted to psychiatric hospital having gone manic again. This time on lithium. Father never takes time off when mum's ill and I had to go. She was managed very badly as a patient as she was a doctor's wife and never really treated by outside doctors. I feel very responsible about helping solve the problem. I had a psychiatry exam too.*

The quotation above highlights another type of patient that doctors find difficult to treat: another doctor or the relatives of a doctor. Traditionally, they are either over-treated or under-treated. We will discuss this further in Chapter 7.

Medicine is an emotionally demanding job and this is sometimes somewhat swept under the carpet. Some stressors will be chronic and so need to be dealt with by long-term solutions to ease or prevent them happening; others will be one-offs that will not usually be possible to plan for and so will need to be tackled after the event. For example:

- **Making mistakes.** Medicine is clearly made much more difficult with the growth of litigation that is sweeping the western world. All doctors find that if they have to face claims or complaints or discipline, this is one of the most difficult times of all in their careers. However, even if there is no complaint, even if a mistake goes largely or wholly unnoticed, doctors still remember them for most of their lives and most doctors have at least one of these tucked away in their memories, one that resurfaces from time to time when things get tough. A specialist trainee wrote:

I missed the diagnosis of pulmonary embolism and treated the patient as a case of severe pneumonia until the day after. Her condition deteriorated and only then was the diagnosis put right. I felt guilty and lost confidence.

It's very human to make mistakes, and they are bound to happen in a difficult job like medicine, so often filled with uncertainty and where advances are happening at a rate of knots. But throughout their careers, whether junior or senior, doctors feel great and lasting shame and distress from where things went wrong. How you tackle those mistakes – the way you use them to learn and the way you think about their cause – are important in terms of how you will feel in the future and even how you will develop as a doctor (see Chapters 5 and 6). We will talk about mistakes much more in Chapter 12.

Where emotions run high, as they are bound to do when you deal with such fundamental issues of life and death, blame can sometimes ricochet around when things go wrong. In reality, it's rarely down to one person or another, and almost always involves systems issues. Nevertheless, one of the most stressful aspects of mistakes is where you get the blame for something you feel was not at all your fault. For example:

I was blamed for a mistake about a patient's medication as I'd taken the message from the consultant in the path lab and he'd got it wrong.

At a time like that, getting support from a senior is particularly important:

My consultant sat me down and reassured me what the situation was and how it wouldn't lead to litigation. She relieved all my anxiety.

Consultants rarely understand just how important they are to junior doctors and how much every word they say of blame or praise has an enormous effect on confidence and is remembered for years. GP trainers play the same role in a primary care setting. It is all too easy for them to forget how stressful and lonely it can be on a house call, when the visiting doctor is exposed to clinical and, on occasions, physical risk. Good supportive backup on the phone, with supportive de-brief sessions, can make all the difference.

- **Complaints and litigation.** Perhaps the most stressful happening of all for doctors occurs when a serious complaint takes place, especially if they have to face litigation or the long drawn-out process of coming before a disciplinary body. At times like this they say they feel utterly alone, isolated from colleagues and patient alike, and suicides are sadly not uncommon. Even after they have been fully exonerated by the disciplinary agency – and this is increasing as these organisations take every complaint much more seriously than they used to do – they often continue to feel demolished by the experience and uncertain in their judgments. One senior doctor said: 'I find I check everything over and over now and often go to colleagues to make sure I'm right. I know I'm sending for far more tests than I used to do as well.'

More trivial complaints, even when embedded in a patient's letter of thanks and appreciation, still raise irritation or anger in most doctors who tend to ignore the good points and see the small complaint as an attack upon their competence or dedication. Learning to see the positive, to recognise the good things you do and to deal with the inevitable stress by learning relaxation or meditation and by getting support beyond your family are all essential strategies at a time like this (see Chapter 5). Remember that colleagues, lawyers and medical defence societies can all support you, but get counselling or other professional help if you are feeling really low.

- **A colleague's under-performance.** Another associated stress is where you become aware that a member of your team may be under-performing. They may turn up late for work, not answer the phone or bleep, refuse to come in when you need help with an urgent case, or fail to do any teaching. You know that you have a responsibility for patient safety, as well as a wider professional requirement to express concerns; but you know too that saying something risks the team's cohesion, and also potentially your own reputation and future references.

We were puzzled by the erratic behaviour of a GP colleague, and struggled to know what to do. He came in late quite a bit and seemed distracted. I can't say that the patient care he gave was dangerous or particularly odd, but something wasn't quite right. In the end we had to talk it through with him. It turned out he had financial problems.

1.5 Things change

Beyond these core issues for doctors there are others which appear at particular points in careers. For example, **students and young doctors** report finding senior doctors difficult to deal with and bullying has been reported as widespread in the past.

He shouted at me and threw a packet of X-rays in my face in front of lots of colleagues, just because my consultant has asked me to get a scan arranged.

I took a day off sick and my consultant told me off saying that in her career she had never taken a day off sick!

My GP Trainer always seemed to want to pick on me. However much I knew, it was never enough. We used to meet up with the nursing and office staff at coffee time, and he would delight in exposing my ignorance to the assembled team.

Such systematic ritual humiliation used to be common practice in many medical teaching settings. That it has not disappeared entirely is a cause for concern, and a reminder that everyone has a responsibility to challenge behaviour that is not acceptable.

In addition, both students and young doctors face examinations and the constant exposure of being evaluated by others and this is never an easy passage. And then there is the new challenge of getting the job they really want in a world where medicine changes regularly from being over- or under-supplied.

Change in itself is at best a challenge and more often very stressful. Although once medicine pottered on with very few drastic changes happening, over the last 20 years successive governments have radically altered the way the health service is organised and how the professions work within it. For doctors this has resulted in a gradual reduction in autonomy. **Senior hospital doctors** used to be the least stressed, but now their levels have risen considerably as the constraints have grown and their roles, particularly in hospitals rather than in general practice, have become more demanding. In addition to those factors we've discussed above, hospital consultants list the following as increasingly stressful:

- Constant change driven from the top;
- Targets that are often meaningless clinically;
- Breakdown of the firm structure;
- Not knowing their junior staff now there is a shift system (tough for the juniors too!);
- Lack of autonomy;
- Bullying managers;
- Too much paperwork;
- The fear of litigation.

GPs, particularly those in partnerships, also face major external pressures which mirror those for senior consultants. The audit culture, with its emphasis on meeting targets and the need to supply endless data on clinical and organisational activity, wears doctors (and their practice managers) down.

I used to think that my job was to meet the needs of my patients. Now it seems that my role is to furnish the Office of National Statistics with endless information of increasingly limited value.

> *Struggling with the need to meet ever changing targets, I am spending much longer in the surgery building, as well as taking paperwork home. As the Senior Partner in a small practice, I worry that the practice income is now falling and that I may have to make some staff redundant.*

One wider challenge to all doctors remains that of the change in the nature of politics, as health care, its costs and organisation, increasingly appears at the centre of the political debate. The emergence of new national strategies and initiatives, such as 'delivery units', and the need for managers and clinicians alike to dance to their political masters' tunes, leave many doctors dismayed and demoralised. In the UK, the historic role of GPs as 'gate keepers' – the expert generalists who guided their individual patients through the system to seek their optimal care and treatment – has to some degree been replaced by a rationing role for the benefit of the wider population. Consultants also feel this pressure to divide their loyalties, aware that the patient in front of them may receive 'second best' treatment for reasons of cost, and knowing that this thought is also in the patient's mind. The mutual respect and trust they both seek is put at risk when talk of rationing and the need to balance budgets takes over.

> *I struggle with how to face the patient's family. They want to know that everything possible is being done, and I want that too. How do I explain that the best chemo option is not on the protocol and that the local Primary Care Trust won't pay for it?*

1.6 Conclusion

It is clear from the above that the context and the time in which you work, and the policies that are introduced or in place at different points are all going to affect both what you see as stressful and your stress levels. To some extent this is going to make it harder for older doctors who have been trained differently and who have had to make many more changes during their careers, than for young doctors who may have fewer expectations and whose new training may make it easier, for example, to work with the patient rather than simply for the patient.

You may feel now that a chapter full of difficulties, as this has been, is enough to distress anyone, but we hope this isn't the case. Rather, it is usually a relief to find that the things you were experiencing as stressful are shared by thousands of others. The good news is that stress levels are clearly changeable to some extent by changing the context in which you work. Ways to handle the distress caused will be discussed in more detail in Part 2.

Bibliography

British Medical Association. *Stress and the Medical Profession*. 1992, BMA, London.

Carter AJ, West MA. Sharing the burden: teamwork in health care settings. In Firth-Cozens, J & Payne, R (eds) *Stress in Health Professionals: Psychological and Organizational Causes and Interventions*. 1999, J. Wiley & Son Ltd, Chichester.

Editorial. The doctor is unwell. *The Lancet* 1993;**342**:1249–50.

Firth-Cozens J. Depression in doctors. In Katona, C & Robertson, MM (eds), *Depression and Physical Illness*. 1997 (pp. 95–111), Wiley, Chichester.

Firth-Cozens J. A perspective on stress and depression. In Cox J, et al. (eds) *Understanding Doctors' Performance*. 2005, Radcliffe Publishing, Oxford.

Firth-Cozens J & Payne R. *Stress in Health Professionals: Psychological and Organizational Causes and Interventions*. J. Wiley & Son Ltd. Wiley's are at Chichester.

Gabe J, et al. *Challenging Medicine*. 1994, Routledge, London.

Harrison, J and van Zwanenberg, T. *GP Tomorrow*. 2002, Radcliffe Publishing, Oxford.

Smith R. Why are doctors so unhappy? *BMJ* 2001;**322**:1073–4.

Chapter 2 **Why me?**

Organisations change and what is a good place to work one year might be a difficult one the next, especially if major upheavals are taking place: mergers and redundancies, new policies and new chief executives will all affect staff at every level. However, there is no doubt that some people show greater resilience to these changes and manage to sail through them apparently unscathed. Even in poor organisations and teams some people survive much better than others. What you generally find in large-scale longitudinal surveys is that there are three groups of people: those who are consistently resilient to most of what life throws at them; those who are affected by particular negative events but fine in most situations; and those who find themselves stressed in a number of organisations, a variety of situations, different teams, perhaps different specialties. They are the ones who, looking around at colleagues who seem to be doing OK despite the difficulties, will ask 'Why me'? In this chapter we are going to look at the individual factors – personality and experiences – that can create temporary or longer-term problems or protect you from them.

2.1 Life events

There are a number of reasons why someone might be more vulnerable either at particular times in their lives or in a number of situations. Life events – the things that happen to you beyond the mundane – have been shown to affect individuals, both physically and mentally. Life events have been given scores, and many of those that hurt us most are negative and involve loss. Although each individual sees events differently, the really big ones that affect most of us are:

- Death of a spouse/partner,
- Divorce,

- Separation,
- Death of a close relative,
- Personal injury or illness,
- Being fired,
- Family illness,
- Financial problems.

Jack came to a coaching session because his senior had suggested to him rather strongly that this might be a good idea. He was clearly very reluctant, made little eye contact and was frowning and tight-lipped; angry, and his anger was getting in the way of a number of previously good relationships. There was a suspicion that he was drinking too much as well. His leg was in a pot, the result of a skiing accident. When he gradually started to talk about his life at the moment, the coach began to note down his life events: a broken leg, negative equity, the end of a relationship, his mother's diagnosis of breast cancer – and all in the last year. On top of that he had his newly experienced work problems: used to being a bit of a star, he now had a boss he didn't seem to get on with, a difficult group of nurses who appeared to have it in for him, too much to do, and so on. All these relationship problems might have been true, or they may have been the result of his own behaviour, his irritable manner, his trouble concentrating, and so on. If anyone has life events, they are likely to be affected emotionally and sometimes physically. Jack was, not surprisingly, depressed as a result of what had been happening to him, and he covered his depression with anger. Like alcohol, anger is a reasonably effective way in the short term to stop yourself feeling so wretched, but not at all useful in the long run: bad for your relationships and not so good for your heart either. Just recognising how much had been happening to him and starting to express his feelings about these events let him make a start on learning new ways to approach the problem and improve his work relationships.

Even some apparently small things can push up your life events score: having a row at work or at home, losing a pet, moving house, having a baby, failing an exam, getting married. You probably know what they say: never move jobs at the same time as you move house, especially if you've just had a baby and it's Christmas.

When someone has experienced a life event – particularly one of those listed above – chances are they will be affected by it to some extent, and others in the team need to recognise this and step in to support them till things are getting better. When someone is behaving badly who usually behaved well, the first question to ask is whether something distressing has happened to him or her. If it happens to you, you need to be as open as you can with at least one person in the team so they can understand and can support you when you need it. The section on emotional intelligence (see below) is relevant to this.

Life events happen to everyone and will affect most people temporarily. Even so, sometimes the event is similar to a previous unpleasant or traumatic experience and this seems to add on to its impact. So health care staff who worked with the victims of the Omagh bombing suffered longer and more severely if they had also been involved in the Enniskillen bombing years earlier. Trauma seems to make an imprint which can be reawakened by similar events. Seneca's comment that 'Time heals what reason cannot' is not always true, neither emotionally nor even physically. For example, marital strife has been shown to cause physical wounds to heal more slowly. Similarly, in a longitudinal study of over 300 doctors, the three students whose mothers had died when they were young became seriously depressed when they started their first house jobs. Numbers are far too small to make any conclusions here, but other studies have suggested similar findings. This doesn't mean that, if your mother died while you were at school you should avoid being a doctor – far from it – but it does suggest that you should recognise that you might need some extra support at times, as most of us do.

2.2 Looking for patterns

Although life events have a temporary impact for most people, a sizable proportion of us find ourselves stressed without extra external events happening – just with the usual aspects of the workplace and the individuals that we interact with. They might feel bullied in a number of different situations, or be told they are bullying themselves. They may find they get angry and in trouble not just in one team but in three or four; that, despite changing specialties to one which seemed easier, they still seem to be getting overloaded and missing deadlines. They may consistently blame themselves for things that go wrong in their lives, or blame others each time something goes amiss. Human beings may be quirky in lots of ways, but they are consistently quirky: consistency of behaviour, of emotions, reactions and attitudes is remarkably high. However, this doesn't mean that people can't change: they can. Once they understand themselves, they can use their strengths to overcome any weaknesses; they can learn ways to change their mood; they can be helped to leave traumas and unhappy relationships behind them. People who abuse drugs and alcohol can use a variety of methods finally to stop destroying their lives. Those who find they end up in the same bad working relationships can be shown why certain personalities clash and how to handle tricky situations. Consistency is what happens when you do nothing to alter the course of your life; change happens when you do.

2.3 Early experience

Our early family experience affects our present relationships in many ways, both in and out of the workplace, and some of these will be developed throughout the book. It may be that a parent was particularly critical or demanding of you and that has made you self-critical or a perfectionist, two characteristics which can cause problems in medicine (see below). In fact, there are studies which show that people in the helping professions as a whole, and especially in certain categories such as mental health and child health, often had particularly difficult childhood experiences themselves. It has been suggested that they go into their careers as a way of trying to resolve the early problems. As this is largely impossible, events in the workplace can be seen as failures, similar to their feelings as a child, and this can be depressing. Similarly, as we said above, people who have experienced early losses in their lives may find adult loss particularly difficult, whether of people close to them or even of some patients.

Insight into these problems and their links to the present usually manage to change their effects for the better. Most of us have imperfect childhoods, and most of us do manage to resolve the issues they create for us as adults, whether through talking to friends, relatives, reading novels, self-help books or occasionally visiting a counsellor. But if they continue and if they are colouring your relationships in a negative way, then longer-term psychotherapy should be considered. Many of the sections below will help you to understand some of the ways that early problems are played out later but can be understood and changed.

2.4 Is gender an issue?

Things are changing in medicine as the proportion of women doctors increases rapidly in most countries. Most articles talk about the workforce issues this is going to pose since women have babies and also are usually still the most responsible for childcare. A few studies have reported that women doctors are more stressed than men, but most find similar levels and longitudinal studies suggest that women doctors' depression levels are mainly predicted by the workplace rather than by any inherently individual problems. There are no differences in general practice, but depression levels rise for some female hospital doctors. Certainly they used to face more difficulties in terms of stereotyping and specialty paths which gave

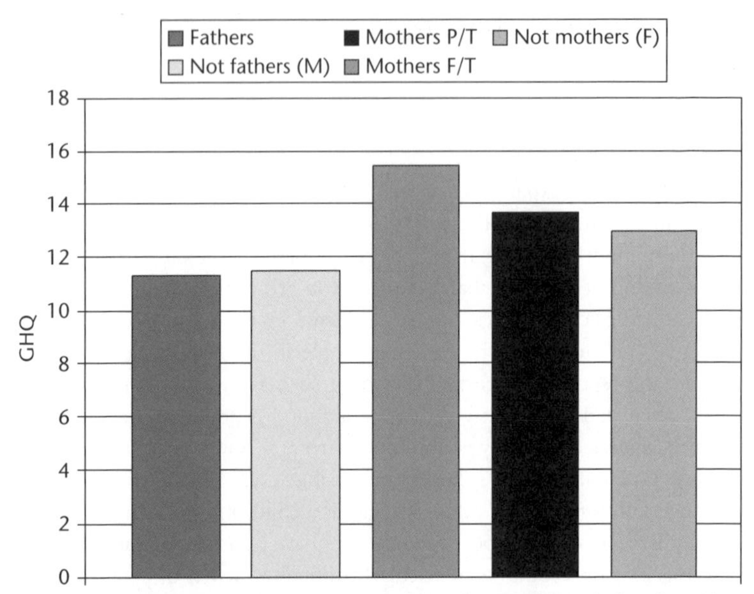

Figure 2.1 Proportions scoring above threshold on the GHQ for male/females with and without children, full time and part time.
(Firth-Cozens J, Redfern N. & Bonanno D (1999). *What is training like? Views on training and support for full-time and flexible specialist registrars.* Report to Northern Postgraduate Deanery of Medicine, Newcastle.)

almost no possibility of family life; and they consistently married less often than men, so perhaps had less social support. In what used to be a very masculine profession, understanding was often hard to find as this young doctor tells us.

> *I recently lost my first baby at 37 weeks. I had just begun my maternity leave and at the end of the three months I was going to take up a consultant's job. My first horrified thought when they told me the baby was dead was: 'Will that mean I have to go back to being a senior registrar?' My consultant rang me the next day to ask if I'd now be able to do a locum, and the hospital personnel officer became irritable and said he'd not had to deal with this before and it was going to be very complicated.*

That's from 20 years ago, and we hope things have changed for the better. Certainly, there are no particular problems for those working in general practice. Nevertheless, from a study of specialty trainees, the group which appears to suffer most are those with children working full time. As you can see from Figure 2.1 for hospital doctors, having children makes no discernible differences to the stress levels of the men!

2.5 Emotional intelligence

Emotional intelligence rose to prominence through the work of Daniel Goleman who put together a considerable amount of research whose results were not always easy to explain. Primarily, it arose from the findings that a proportion of university students with particularly high IQs, like most of you, who should eventually find themselves enjoying excellent jobs and a good life, often ended up (in terms of salary, status, life satisfaction and good relationships) no better and sometimes worse on a number of criteria than students with much lower IQs. Something happened to them which made them blow it, one way or another.

There are several illustrations of this within medicine itself. In the 1970s a new medical school began in Newcastle, New South Wales. One of its founding ideals was to provide more doctors who would be prepared to work in outback towns or those without the glamour and high-flyer credentials of Sydney. They decided to try a new approach to selection and so chose students for their problem-solving, their empathy, their integrity, rather than simply their intellectual abilities. However, around half the students were still selected in the old way, as they were in the cities, based mainly on academic achievements. They found that, at the end of the five years, there was no difference in the levels of success in either group, and so they began to select all their students by the new method. On follow-up years later they found their students had higher job satisfaction and reported greater quality of life than those from the older universities. It seems that IQ might not mean as much as we think in terms of success and life satisfaction.

Much more recently studies of doctors who come up before disciplinary boards have looked back at how these doctors behaved when they were students. They show that problems at medical school – getting drunk, becoming depressed, having trouble with others – were greater in this group than in controls. These studies have led to many medical schools deciding to keep much more careful assessments of students that will be carried on throughout their careers. In case this seems too Orwellian, the idea is that students or young doctors who have such problems will be offered help then and there, so that they do not go on to experience more serious difficulties that threaten their later careers. What these people with high IQs need to learn is emotional intelligence or EQ.

With a large amount of similar evidence along the lines that IQ isn't everything, researchers in the field vary in their definitions of EQ, but largely agree that it consists of the ability to

- perceive emotion in others and in yourself – that is, perceptive skills and self-awareness;
- use this emotional information well to promote thought and reasoning;
- manage your emotions well, even negative ones, to achieve your goals.

Some theorists suggest these are abilities which can be taught; others describe them as traits, which can also be altered, but less easily. The ability to recognise and use emotions well in yourself will often grow with experience; others will need some form of psychotherapy to be able to learn how to give names to what they are feeling, how these feelings affect their perceptions and behaviour, and how to manage them better. The section on the Myers Brigg Type Inventory (MBTI)® below and the chapters on stress management (Chapter 5) and anger (Chapter 8) will help in this regard.

2.6 Self-criticism and perfectionism

Self-criticism, even when measured as students, is one of the main predictors of later depression in doctors over some decades – so it matters. It's not that self-critical doctors (and there are lots of them) are open about whatever they see as their problems – they don't go round owning up to everything – but more that it gives them sleepless nights worrying about what people think of them, thinking they're not good enough, not likeable and so on. This can make them quite irritable, defensive and even aggressive with others as they see blame or criticism even when it is not implied, so colleagues will sometimes view them as very touchy.

Self-criticism is particularly high in psychiatrists and some GPs, and very low in surgeons. If doctors are rarely self-critical they are much less likely to become stressed or depressed but, because they are more likely to see negative events as due to external forces (colleagues, the X-ray department, the partner,

Ian, a GP in his mid-50s, always worried that his clinical knowledge was weak and that patients thought he was a poor doctor, despite his popularity in filling his appointment slots quickly and receiving positive patient feedback. Recently he became anxious about completing his appraisal forms and preparing for future revalidation. Issues came to a head because the daughter of one of his patients made a complaint against him. As a result he felt quite wretched and considered resigning from the practice and taking his pension early. He shared this with his practice manager. Together they offered to meet the daughter with a conciliator to talk through the family's concerns. Ian also sought help from a local confidential counselling service for doctors. The other doctors in the practice valued Ian's clinical advice, although they found him difficult at times because of his obsessional tendencies over following practice protocols. However, they were clear now that they needed to support him more directly while he dealt with the complaint, and agreed to remove some of his paperwork burdens (even though some were self-induced).

the equipment, the patient), it is not uncommon for their colleagues and relatives to suffer from elevated stress levels in dealing with the blame and sometimes the bullying that comes with very low self-criticism.

Perfectionism is a related characteristic that can cause or be a sign of psychological problems. It is sometimes linked to obsessional traits (so common in young doctors as to be almost an occupational hazard), and is usually seen as a sign of anxiety: the world will fall apart if everything isn't completely and utterly perfect. Again, this can cause poor relationships in the workplace, since perfection is usually expected of others as well as oneself, and can also cause problems because of slowness and irritability. Because as a perfectionist you are setting yourself up for constant failure, it can eventually lead to depression.

Being self-critical or a perfectionist might sound good to patients but, as you see, they are not ideal for the doctor. What you are aiming for is a 'good enough' doctor, rather than one who *always* blames himself or herself when something goes wrong instead of thinking about all the things that might have contributed to what's happened – some to do with you perhaps, but also some to do with the context or other people (see Chapter 12 on mistakes) – so that you can learn more fully from the incident. Tackling your thoughts, as we suggest in Chapters 5 and 6, and by learning a little self-compassion rather than being harsh on yourself constantly will help. Practising relaxation or meditation or any of the stress-reducing techniques will support you in tackling the anxiety you might feel when you decide to let things go in a less than perfect state.

2.7 The MBTI™

The MBTI is a psychological assessment of your preferences for the way you are in life. It is not a test of what you can do, but a description of what you prefer doing and how you feel most comfortable doing it. So, if you are right-handed you would rather sign your name with that hand, but if you break your wrist you will soon quite easily sign with your left, despite preferring to use your right. The MBTI, based on Jung's typology, was developed further to look at how people learnt, but is now the most used assessment in organisations around the world – not for selection but for encouraging a valuing of differences, helping people work together and understanding different strengths, so it's particularly useful for team development. At some point in your careers – as early as you can – you should be offered the opportunity to find out your type because it will allow you to make much more sense of the relationships in your working environment and at home, and how to manage them better. The description of the four dimensions in Table 2.1 will give you some idea of your type and there are a number of

Table 2.1 Description of the four dimensions

Introversion (I): Is work out their decision-making in their heads and use privacy to recharge their batteries. They think first, speak later and largely prefer small groups to large noisy gatherings.	**Extraversion (E):** Es work out their decisions by talking to others and use others to recharge their batteries. They tend to speak first, think later and can be attuned to conversations around them as well as their own.
Sensing (S): Ss are observant, realistic, practical, good at details. They live in the present but value the past.	**Intuition (N):** Ns use hunches and gut feelings. They are future oriented, imaginative and into the big picture rather than detail. They like change and variety. They work in bursts of enthusiasm.
Thinking (T): Ts make their decisions according to rationality and logic. They are good at critical analysis, speak their minds and take criticism well themselves. Conflict is not unpleasant to them but they want to get to the bottom of it.	**Feeling (F):** Fs are 'people people'. They are tactful and encouraging and dislike conflict. Harmony matters most. They decide with their hearts rather than their heads. They are subjective and can be greatly hurt by criticism.
Judging (J): Js prefer to live decisively, in a structured, planned manner and like things organised. They have a strong work ethic and are good at lists and prioritising. They like finishing things and making decisions.	**Perceiving (P):** Ps don't like final decisions, preferring to think of them as provisional. They are not keen on finishing things – a deadline is a signal to start work. They are flexible and spontaneous and like to keep options open.

books (see the bibliography) which will go into it in some very useful detail, but a full assessment will always be best.

When you do the assessment you end up with a type made up of four letters, such as ENTP or ISFJ. An understanding of the differences allows you to make sense of why some people irritate you more than others – Js will find very frustrating the inability of Ps to make final decisions or to pack their bags in plenty of time; while Ps may find Js' speed of decision-making sometimes means that important options have been overlooked, or that pleasant time has been wasted by having to get to the airport so early. Es may find that they misconstrue the silence of Is as being negative or obstinate, whereas they only want to think about it. Is may find Es very noisy and intrusive. Fs can find Ts hyper-critical and always pushing for an argument; while Ts can find negative feedback from an F impossible to follow as it is couched in such pleasant language. Ss will see Ns as never attending to the detail and always thinking of new ideas, while Ns might find Ss as too much lodged in the past to plan well for the future. The important thing about this is that all these dimensions, at both sides of the divide, are vitally important in the workplace and at home – people are simply different but need to be valued for their strengths while appreciating their weaknesses.

We shall use these dimensions frequently throughout the book – for example, in career choice, long-term relationships and getting on with difficult people – so you may find it useful to refer back to them frequently or to develop your understanding through one of the recommended books.

2.8 Summary

All these individual quirks, traits and experiences are going to influence the way you perceive various events at work – whether you find some of them stressful or whether they have little effect upon you. In the next part of the book we shall look at ways of dealing with difficult aspects of your career.

Bibliography

Brewin CR, Firth-Cozens J. Dependency and self-criticism as predicting depression in young doctors. *J Occup Health* (APA) 1997;**2**:3, 242–6.

Clack GB, Allen J, Cooper D, Head J. Personality differences between doctors and their patients. *Med Educ* 2004;**38**:177–86.

Cox J, et al. *Understanding Doctors' Performance*. 2005. Radcliffe, Oxford.

Firth-Cozens J. Depression in doctors. In Katona, C & Robertson, MM (eds) *Depression and Physical Illness*. 1997 (pp. 95–111), Wiley, Chichester.

Firth-Cozens J. The psychological problems of doctors. In Firth-Cozens, J & Payne, R (eds) *Stress in Health Professionals: Psychological and Organizational Causes and Interventions*. J. Wiley & Son Ltd. Wiley's are at Chichester.

Goleman D. *Emotional Intelligence: Why It Can Matter More Than IQ*. 1996, Bloomsbury, London.

Kroeger O. *Type Talk at Work*. 1992, Tilden Press, New York.

Newman M. *Emotional Capitalists: The New Leaders*. 2008, John Wiley & Sons, Chichester.

Part 2 Waving, not drowning

Chapter 3 **You and your partner: for life?**

Long-term partnerships (LTPs),[1] whether they involve a marriage or not, are good for you. This was particularly true for men, but now it seems both sexes have better mental and physical health in a good long-term relationship. However, first- and second-time marriages are declining and divorce is increasing. As we saw earlier, separation and divorce are major life events, always enough to throw you off course for a while in some way, often in the workplace; bad for both of you and very sad and disturbing for your children. This is true for everyone, not just doctors.

Nevertheless, the divorce rates for doctors are high. The Johns Hopkins' Precursors Study, a large-scale longitudinal study that followed doctors graduating from 1944 to 1960, found a cumulative incidence of divorce of 29% with wide differences between the different specialties. Marrying before graduation increased the risk – better to wait till life gets a bit more settled, it seems. While 22–24% of paediatricians and pathologists divorced, 33% of surgeons and an enormous 50% of psychiatrists did so: very high rates for couples of that generation who were undoubtedly more conservative than those who followed. This chapter describes the difficulties that may emerge in long-term relationships, whether opposite sex or same sex.

3.1 Work–home balance in medicine

Work–home balance has suffered for many people over the last few decades; for doctors it has always been a major problem. In a longitudinal study of UK doctors, the conflict between work and personal life was seen as one of the top four stressors over 20 years for both men and women. Years of training, long

[1]We will call all LTPs as short hand for the variety of committed partnerships that can exist between two people, while "divorce" refers to any permanent separation.

hours, insufficient sleep, moving around for jobs, examinations – none of it is really conducive to a stable family life. Although the divorce rate for doctors nowadays may be more similar to those in the general population, there is some evidence that their LTPs may be less happy than those of others.[2] Lasting conflict within an LTP is very bad emotionally for you both and any children you may have. In fact, it's likely to affect you physically too: even wounds have been found to heal more slowly in people experiencing marital strife!

Until quite recently, most doctors were men, and of those men who married, half were married to nurses (who were almost always women). This allowed a particular form of symbiosis, not least if the work model of relationship between doctors and nurses transferred into the domestic setting. Equally, the wives of GPs often became subsumed into the GP practice – as nurses, practice managers or by answering the telephone at nights and weekends. This further blurred the definition of where and what was 'work' and what was 'home'.

As more women entered the medical workforce, doctors became more likely to marry other doctors, rather than nurses, with the added pressure of planning and managing two medical careers. Should the woman choose a hospital speciality and the man general practice, this may add a further dimension in relation to perceived status within the medical hierarchy (hospital medicine has more prestige) and the flexibility of training options as there are more variety of possibilities for GP training. Same sex partnerships offer very similar challenges to heterosexual relationships.

In heterosexual relationships, several studies have found that women doctors have a higher divorce rate than men. With the rise in the proportion of women training as doctors, the risk of divorce may increase where the woman is seen as having a status superior to her husband, especially when he is not a doctor. If they are both doctors, whose career takes precedence when other cities or countries beckon one or other for that better job? These tensions between the sexes may officially be out of date, and many couples have overcome them successfully; however, they still remain an issue.

Moreover, as we saw in Chapter 2, women doctors with children working full time in hospital medicine are by far the most stressed and depressed of the sexes, while children seem to make little difference at all to the stress symptoms of men, despite any conflicts they might perceive. There is no doubt from this and other studies just who it is who carries the emotional weight of family life in most marriages; in fact, full-time women doctors have been found to have almost full responsibility for running the family and the home. There's no getting away from the fact that the pressures of both work and home life, whether it includes children or not, are often more

[2]Gabbard & Menninger, *JAMA* 1989.

difficult for women: they can stay without a partner, they can have a partner and have a greater chance of divorce than male doctors, they can remain childless, or they can have children and risk much higher levels of stress, especially if they continue to work full time in hospital medicine. Difficult choices, especially for women who do not want to be GPs where there are no gender differences in stress or depression levels.

So being a doctor can make it more difficult to maintain a happy LTP, which means you probably have to work harder to enjoy the benefits this may bring. There will be some things about the workplace, and the hours you keep, that you can change for the better, and many of the chapters in this book offer solutions for doing that. Nevertheless, it's always a good idea to reflect on what contribution you yourself might be making to any problems in the relationship. If it's a question of whether it's your job or your partner or you causing most of the problems, then the only thing you can be sure of changing is you. What follows is an outline of some of the individual reasons for why things can go wrong, with implications of how to improve them.

3.2 Being different

The Myers Brigg types described in Chapter 2 are very important for understanding some of the things that go wrong in marriages. There are obvious differences when one of you is an I (Introvert), like most hospital doctors, and the other is an E (Extrovert), like most GPs, but these can usually be easily overcome with a little understanding and some give-and-take around your social lives. The only more serious relationship challenge will come if there are other problems since Is find it more difficult to discuss them. In this case, the partner who is an E has to provide more quiet space to let the I partner talk. Men find talking about their feelings much more difficult than women do anyway, so if the man is also an I – and especially if both of you are Is – then there may be a lot of things unsaid which would be better out in the open. See the exercises at the end of the chapter to help you find ways of expressing them.

If you differ in the Intuitive–Sensing (N–S) dimension, this too is unlikely to prove problematic if you use the differences well. For example, the S will probably be good at attending to the detail and the here-and-now, while the N will be useful on the planning side, providing several alternatives for things and thinking up new possibilities. If he or she is also a P (Perception), then this process might go on for an irritatingly long time as Ps tend to enjoy playing with alternatives rather than making a decision. This is particularly frustrating to a J (Judgment) partner who likes to get things organised and finished in plenty of time. A J will want to pack for a holiday days or even weeks in advance, while a P will be happy to throw a few things into a suitcase at the last minute. But Ps can be organised – it's going to be essential in all their work – and Js can be spontaneous and wait, not too impatiently, until they're sure the right decision has been made. Acting the opposite of your type can actually be quite fun, at least for a short while, and gives you a whole new perspective on how to live your life.

These are very ordinary differences – sometimes irritating, but unlikely to lead to real animosity. The dimension that can affect relationships deeply if understanding is lacking is the T–F (Thinking–Feeling) dimension, because when one of you is a T and the other is an F you are likely to feel you need very different levels of appreciation and you may imagine you have fundamentally different values. As we saw in Chapter 2, an F is careful with the feelings of others, wants them to be careful of his or her feelings, wants to be appreciated generally, hates conflict and has person-centred values which reflect these relationship issues. A T, on the other hand, is blunt, can even appear tactless, needs less appreciation and primarily only from those they admire, and has values that depend on issues of justice and rationality rather than relationships. In medicine, feedback, appreciation and values are core to everyday work. At the end of a tiring and emotionally demanding day, an F may report to a T partner that she or he is upset by something taken as poor feedback from her junior, or by a patient who was rude and unappreciative. The partner may feel the same stress from the day, but for different reasons – that the workload had been unequally or unfairly organised, or the senior partner had criticised their time-keeping when really it was the fault of the practice manager. The T shows no obvious appreciation of the meal cooked by the F and they begin to argue over the level at which health care rationing should be achieved and whether the birthday card F sent to an elderly patient was really the right thing for a doctor to do.

You can see that this dimension can cause the sort of problems that make a couple feel they have nothing at all in common. But we promise you that, once you understand that you are simply different and appreciate what this makes the other one feel, then you can begin to work on how to change your behaviours somewhat towards those that the other partner expects. So a T can become tactful and less critical (really, we can learn to keep our mouths tight shut at times) and can practise appreciation of others; while an F can realise that straight statements are a reflection of T's honesty rather than criticism or nastiness, and that there is a limit to how much interacting they can expect (especially if the T is also an Introvert!), and that being rational about the provision of medicine doesn't mean that T does not want the best for his or her patients.

Understanding Type can be one of the best means of partnership therapy you can undertake, and it will also be good for any children you may have.

An Introverted little boy in a big noisy family of Extroverts can sometimes be judged abnormal or even neurotic, rather than simply different; while a single SJ daughter, with her eye for detail and organisation, can find herself responsible for all the administrative household chores the rest of the family finds too boring because they are all NPs. Start thinking about yourselves in Type terms, and you will begin to appreciate difference, enjoy it, and even try some of the skills and strengths of your opposite.

3.3 Being self-centred

In order to achieve what you have done, you've had to focus on yourself for a long, long time. Your social life might have been riotous, but that too can leave less time for the development of the skills needed to build a good relationship. Moreover, you spend your working hours participating in the care of others, and this will make some people less able to provide the type of nurture necessary for an LTP. Why should you come home and be expected to give even more? If you marry another doctor, then this might be the coming together of two people who are primarily used to the world existing only round them and who have not yet had the practice of entering that space between where you can meet and enjoy each other and be creative of something that will last.

The first cure for this is recognition – might this be happening to you? This is an area where insight can be very powerful in terms of change. Ask yourself:

- How often do I notice my partner – what they are wearing, what they are reading, whether they look tired, content, sad? Try doing it.
- How often do I talk to him or her about the day? About the garden, the holiday, the children? Not just the problems, but the good things too?
- How often do the two of you go out together where talk is not important – walking, a concert, a gallery?

If one of you is an E and the other is an I, then what appears as self-centredness to the I may just be that Es talk a lot more and that people very quickly know all about them. If you are an E, then do remember that Is need a little peace and quiet and, if they are also Fs, they might like you to ask about them too.

3.4 The competition for power

Most doctors feel some power in the workplace, and some experience it in heaps. If one or both of you take that power-surge into the home, then there can be trouble. You must have been reasonably competitive to have got as far as you have, and competitiveness too is fine in most situations – but not at home. Power is rarely equal in a marriage, but also it can shift over time so even if you're top dog now, you might not be later in the relationship. Again, it's only by looking honestly at how you use your power that will help to ensure that you use it well. If you discover that you always want to win, let your partner win instead and see how it feels. If you find it feels very demoralising, then you need to do it more often!

In Myers Brigg terms, Ts, with their liking for strong debate can sometimes come across as very competitive to an F, and maybe this is right but, more likely, they just love the to-and-fro of what Fs might see as a conflict. If you are a T and feel the need to impose your views or even your will, you should try giving your partner a hug instead!

3.5 The problem solver

Another form of power involves the desire to sort out problems, especially those belonging to other people. Problem-solving is a key attribute of being a good doctor, which patients, their families and the health service value. However, transferring this skill into the domestic setting can bring its own problems, not least when both parties want to solve a given 'problem' in quite different ways! Also trying to sort out your children's lives is risky. How many offspring of doctors have ended up in medical careers only to find that what worked for their parents doesn't work for them?

Being conscious of the ingrained habit of seeking problems to solve is the first step to self-awareness in this area. Being able to distinguish which problems are soluble and which are not, as well as which are appropriate to engage with, is a sign of maturity, which we will come back to in Chapter 5.

It's possible that both of you fit the mould of competitive problem solvers, in which case you will inevitably lock horns from time to time over the big issues of life – family, finance, where to live, children's school choices and the like. The need to explore how such decisions are to be made, in part through clarifying underlying beliefs and values, is ongoing throughout our lives, not least as we each change over time through the people we meet and the experiences we encounter.

3.6 Personality

Doctors have two dimensions of personality that are different to other professional groups: they are higher on perfectionism and on the obsessional-compulsive dimension. It is hard to know if these are really aspects of personality or whether they reflect something in the job – more a deep fear of making an error and so wanting to check things more carefully and strive to do everything better and better: only perfect is good enough. But perfectionism can cause relationship problems both at work and at home, especially if it leads you to expect others in the family to have the same very high standards and then appearing very critical when they don't. Moreover, perfectionists are more likely to become depressed, especially if they are self-critical, as most are (see Chapters 2 and 6) and depression can be very difficult for LTPs, whether the depressed person is miserable and withdrawn, or whether they are angry and aggressive. The sooner depression is recognised and dealt with, the better for both of you.

Perfectionism may appear to some to be a rather useful trait for doctors to have; however, it is always going to be impossible to achieve and so you will inevitably set yourself up for failure if you expect it. Learn early on to aim reasonably high, but also talk to others about their standards and where you fit in the general run of doctors. Be less self-critical, and more compassionate towards yourself, and you will find you can be kinder to others too. Like everyone else, you will never be perfect, and that is easier to live with if you can get support from colleagues and your partner. To be 'good-enough' is usually good enough.

3.7 Stress and anger

We know from the findings we discussed in the Introduction that proportionally more of you will be stressed and depressed than the general public. This inevitably spills over into your home life. If the stress seems to come from your considerable time pressures, then that is bound to impact doubly upon your relationships: you will show all the usual stress symptoms, including impatience and irritability, and you will probably have less time to talk about them. So you need to address both these issues: first, by making time to talk to your partner about what's happening to you and how you're going to tackle it; and, second, by tackling your stress with some of the ways suggested in Chapter 5, or whatever works for you (other than alcohol and other drugs!). If you and your partner think that it might be depression that is causing the problems, then do consult your GP: don't self-prescribe. Doctors are notoriously bad at looking after their own health (and often not wonderful at caring for their family's health either), but depression will inevitably affect your relationship negatively and needs to be addressed early.

Years of running stress management workshops have shown that irritability and anger are the predominant feature of stress (and often of depression too) in over-stretched staff. Around a quarter of them show this anger at work, another quarter experience it at work *and* at home, and around half show it only at home. When you think about this statistically, it means that, since around a quarter to a third of health care staff are stressed, at least half of these will be making life unpleasant for their colleagues, while a slightly different half will be making things bad at home. In the Precursors Study at Johns Hopkins, doctors who scored in the highest quartile of the anger scale were much more likely to divorce than the rest. In time the anger and the problems it causes at home will reverberate on the workplace, and vice versa. It's not surprising that so many of our organisations and some of our homes are far from the sociable, productive and fulfilling places they could be. Because anger is such a destructive force in a relationship and at work, there is a separate chapter (Chapter 8) on this emotion and exercises on how to tackle it, but here is one for the two of you.

> ***Dealing with the everyday:*** One way to nip anger in the bud is to tell each other daily what you appreciated the other one doing or saying, and what you resented them doing or saying. These things can be as large or as small as you like – small is great, in fact. So, 'I appreciated you for bringing me a cup of tea' or '...for asking me about my day', or '...dealing with the plumber yourself'. On the other hand, 'I resented you for dropping your towels on the bathroom floor', or '...telling the children I would tell them off', or '...saying that I always rub people up the wrong way'. This doesn't just stop you building small resentments into bigger ones, it also provides a stroke of appreciation that is often absent in busy relationships.

3.8 Things happen

If we're talking about a long-term relationship we're talking about decades. Things will happen during those years, and people will change, often not in the ways that you wanted them to. Children arrive, adolescents are difficult, spouses retrain, parents get ill or die, children leave home. All these things are difficult and all of them affect the individual partners and their relationship. At times one or other will feel unappreciated, unloved, scared of aging, fed up with the humdrum, frightened to change. But dealing with change is a large part of what life, including life together, is all about. As the Buddhists say – this is it.

There are particularly tricky periods in all LTPs. In the first few years you're working out how to get along together, especially if you have new children and new jobs. In the mid-life women often become more assertive, which might be difficult for some men. Men, on the other hand, often become more intimate, and not always with their partners. Mid-life crises happen to both sexes, to men somewhat earlier than women. These crises are very often really a form of depression, or an ill-conceived means of warding off depression. They come at a time when parents are aging and mortality is glimpsed for them and so also for you; adolescent children are becoming difficult and assertive; your partner's looks aren't what they were. You haven't achieved everything at work that you dreamed of, and now you know you won't. Men in particular find it easy to leap on quick-fix solutions – nice sports car, toupee, trendy clothes, and a new younger partner – and to see every reason why the first marriage was a mistake – 'I grabbed the first hand I could as soon as I graduated;' 'I thought a nurse would look after me'; 'Our marriage was never good'; 'Sex was always bad'. But those words 'always' and 'never' are very unlikely to be true, and the good parts of that relationship as well as its offspring are well worth hanging onto, at least for a time while you cool down from your ardour and get help in trying to mend your relationship, especially if children are involved. One of the most unfortunate phrases of the last few decades is 'Children are resilient'. They're not, and divorce causes them great pain and consequences that, for some, last throughout their lives.

Affairs are always painful, but for the hurt partner – the one who didn't have the affair – forgiveness and trust are rarely impossible with time, and it's usually a shame to throw away everything because of a single transgression. Hospital environments in particular are over-heated in all sorts of ways – as Freud told us, *thanatos* and *eros*, death and sex, are often enmeshed. But it's very painful to feel tricked, lied to, unappreciated and unloved at times

Last month Maria learnt that her husband Joe had been having an affair. He'd told his best friend who had told his wife when they were having a row, and then she's told Maria. It was bound to leak back, but people often want to be found out. She knew things hadn't been good and that they had drifted apart each with their full-time work, and the children being difficult now they were teenagers, but she still felt devastated. When she confronted him he admitted it but said it was over. She believed him, but wanted to talk about it – the details of the affair and what they as a couple were going to do to make things better between them. But he wouldn't talk about it. She found she got more upset and untrusting by this – could she believe him at all? – but she got him to go for couples counselling. There they did various exercises such as writing lists of what had first attracted them to each other and how they could capture that again; agreeing to daily appreciations and resentments (which he found difficult but managed as it was structured rather than emotional), and Maria realised that there was no point looking for something called The Truth over the affair, because whatever she was told she might never fully believe. Better to start again from today. It took time, but things gradually got better as they kept up the exercises and left the pain behind.

like this, so take time to let yourself heal and to find ways of overcoming what, over the lifetime of a long relationship, can often shrink to a pinprick rather than a fatal stabbing.

Like much in medicine, prevention is better than cure. Spending regular amounts of time at work with others, whether doctors, non-medical staff, or patients in a GP setting, increases the risk of an inappropriate liaison developing. This should act as a warning, not least in relation to matters of medical licensing where patients are concerned. The wise course is to be aware of the dangers, and not think that it happens only to others – that somehow I am immune from such risks and temptations when others are not.

3.9 Recipe for the long term

If you want to avoid problems in your relationship, or do something about those that are developing, here are a few key strategies for you to follow:

- Don't think you and your partner can mind-read. Better to carve out regular times to talk together, so problems don't escalate.
- Provide daily appreciations and resentments.
- List the things that first brought you together and see what can be done to recapture some of them.
- Seek out frequent opportunities to relax together.
- Work out what you both are in terms of your MBTI Types and think about how this will affect your relationship and how you can use your differences well and enjoy them.
- Allow space for the other to flourish and don't try to solve all his or her problems.
- Attend individually to your stress – learn and practise a form of relaxation (or meditation) and get support or professional help when you need it.
- Don't rush into separating from your partner if things go badly wrong for a while. Get counselling help and appreciate that time really does heal most one-off transgressions.
- Remember that your career puts extra demands on relationships, so you have to work at things just that bit harder. But the rewards for all of you will be worth it.

Bibliography

Cozens J. *To Have and to Hold: Men, Sex and Marriage.* 1995, Pan, London.

Gerber LA. *Married to Their Careers: Career & Family Dilemmas in Doctors' Lives.* 1983, Tavistock Publications, New York.

Pringle R. *Sex and Medicine: Gender, Power and Authority in the Medical Profession.* 1998, Cambridge University Press, Cambridge.

Chapter 4 **Choosing a specialty**

4.1 Why medicine?

It's probable that almost everyone reading this has already chosen to do medicine. It's quite likely too that many of you have at times wondered why on earth you did it, though most doctors are pretty satisfied with their careers eventually. In an interview study, Isobel Allen concluded that the majority had decided on their career path because they'd been good at science, or 'to fulfil the aims and aspirations of others'. Those don't seem to be wonderful reasons and probably most of you thought of other things at times: it's still a prestigious occupation; a parent might have been a doctor; you wanted a good salary and a secure job; or did you just want to help people? There is also some evidence that the choice has some unconscious factors to it, influenced by early events in your lives. For example, one study compared medical students and law students, looking at the number of illnesses and legal problems within their early families and found that medical students were more likely to have experienced illness in the family and law students to have had legal problems. Others have suggested that many helping professionals as a whole are trying to repair something from their early childhood, and this might be an example of that urge to make things good. Whether that also affects specialty choice has yet to be studied.

It can seem strange to outsiders that doctors go through such a long shared training and yet end up in such very different jobs. Just compare a surgeon and a psychotherapist, an emergency physician with a dermatologist, the role of a pathologist and a GP: they're all vastly different occupations. For this reason it has been argued that medicine is a broad church and needs all sorts of people to enter it at undergraduate level. Nevertheless, such different future roles should perhaps require considerable thought, and even professional help, once the time arrives to choose a specialty. If you are going to be happy in your role – and so if your patients are going to be happy with you – requires proper career advice, perhaps psychometrics – at least a series of brief 'taster' experiences of short-listed specialties.

However, career counselling for doctors, advice on why people choose different specialties, and research on what makes a good choice for whom are all still in their infancies. In this chapter we will pull together some of the work and ideas that exist.

4.2 So why choose that?

Given a list of the reasons for entering a particular specialty, the most common factor chosen by all doctors has been that they enjoyed the clinical content that the role entailed – the nature of the job satisfied them. That's good news and suggests that either people choose carefully, perhaps changing specialties once or twice until they are satisfied, or that most people are able to become fascinated by any subject if they study it in depth, really start to understand it and feel good at it. Chances are it's a combination of both factors. However, the reason for starting to get interested in an area in the first place seems greatly influenced by having a good experience of it during your training. If there was an enthusiastic role model who could show you the pleasures and fascinations of that specialty, then you are much more likely to enter it. Unfortunately, this works even more strongly the other way so that, if you have a bad experience in a particular specialty, then this makes a lasting imprint and reminder that you won't go there.

Wanting to work fewer hours – for all sorts of lifestyle reasons – has become less of an issue now that working hours have reduced in many countries. However, it is still a major influence on those with families or those who want less stress. GPs, in particular, choose their careers partly because of wanting more time for children and also because they want more contact with patients, more freedom in practising, and because it fits in better with a partner's job. Public health specialists and laboratory-based doctors have given their main reasons for deciding on their particular specialties as wanting less patient contact and less stress.

4.3 Different specialties and the influence of stress

How stressed you find your first postgraduate years does have an effect on specialty choice: longitudinal studies show that those who were most stressed at that time were more likely to choose specialties which they saw as having less stress, less contact with patients and working fewer hours.

Those with high stress were, sensibly, much less likely to choose careers for reasons of prestige or money. Measured while they were students, many of those with high levels of stress and depression followed one of two routes – some choosing laboratory-based specialties or public health where their patient contact was minimal, and others choosing psychiatry where contact was high and perhaps where they felt they could explore their own problems.

It's clear from this that any stress or depression you experience before you need to choose a career may still be an important influence on your eventual choice. It seems too that the cause of the stress is seen as being quite closely linked to patient contact: for some people, getting close to patients causes more stress rather than less. This is born out by Table 4.1 which comes from a study following doctors from being fourth year students over 17 years to when they became house officers (or interns) and finally senior doctors. The specialty categories are grouped according to how close they want to be to their patients, with general practice and psychiatry at the top and laboratory-based careers and public health medicine at the bottom. The scores are mean scores for the 12-item General Health Questionnaire (GHQ-12), a widely used measure of the emotional distress of different populations.

You can see that the psychiatrists are the most stressed, and this has grown over time. You might feel that this is a result of their jobs, which are difficult and where patient-related rewards are fairly thin on the ground. However, they are also the most stressed group as students, the other being those who later chose laboratory-based careers or public health medicine. This group and those who finally chose anaesthetics or radiology were very stressed in their first postgraduate year but appear to have chosen well so their stress levels have reduced to barely above normal as seniors. Numbers are small, but these findings are replicated in other studies (Table 4.1).

From these studies it seems a good policy, if you are stressed or depressed as a student (and many are) that, first, you should do something about

Table 4.1 Stress levels according to specialty

Specialty	Stress as students	Stress in PGY1	Stress as seniors
General practice	11.5	12.3	12.9
Psychiatrists	13.4	14.3	16.0
General medical	11.5	12.7	11.9
Surgery	10.5	9.5	10.6
Anaesthetics, radiology	13.0	13.3	11.6
Laboratory and Public health medicine	12.7	15.5	11.9

the problem since it may influence your career choice in ways that are not ideal; second, if you don't tackle the problem, then don't choose psychiatry as it will not help your stress levels and may make things worse. Psychiatric patients are perhaps the least appreciative of all, and if you're self-critical (and psychiatrists have the highest scores for this too) it is likely to be a painful process to face each day patients who would often rather not see you at all and resent some of the treatments and support you offer.

The other glaring finding shown in this table is that surgeons are so very, very cheerful! Whether you assess them as students or at any time in their careers, they top the table for wellbeing and job satisfaction. Because these data are longitudinal, again you can see that it's not just the job – it's not only that their patients are extra grateful to them, or that they earn more money or have more status – no, they came that way to the job. So we choose our jobs partly because of our psychological make-up including our mental health. Tackling any problems in this area before you graduate will probably give you a wider choice of specialties, and you can make your decisions for much better reasons.

4.4 Disability

Being physically disabled is not usually a deterrent to being a doctor, and there is little or no stigma from colleagues or from patients. In fact, reports suggest that some patients appear very positive about having a doctor who seems to be in a worse situation to them!

> *In the vast majority, staff and patients alike appear to have no (or few) preconceptions about what I am able to do, and if in doubt will ask if I would like any assistance. I think I meet less discrimination at work than outside (amputee).*

However, it's worth being sensible about what specialty you decide upon. Although most disability discrimination legislation states that 'reasonable adjustments' must be made for disability, you may find that organisational factors can prove a hassle to you over a long period of time – you may have the right to these adjustments but getting them done over and over again can take great determination.

> *The accommodation was supposed to have been adapted before I moved in (things such as tap handles, shower rail, door handles). However, nothing was done even two/three weeks after I had already started work (arthritis).*

> *Going to see a patient and then finding out that the medical notes are too heavy for me to carry. Sometimes there is no one free to help me so I need to wait around until I can ask somebody. (arthritis)*

> *Exposure to anaesthetic agents may make me feel more fatigued. (chronic fatigue)*

Not everyone is suited to every specialty, whether they have a disability or not, so if there is a large part of the role that gives you frequent problems, don't give yourself extra stress and pain by thinking that this is the one route that will let you be happy.

Remember – most people are satisfied with their final career choice once they get into it.

However, doctors with mental health problems – particular bipolar disorders – do sometimes have a more difficult time, both with the nature of their disability and because of factors within training and attitudes of colleagues and patients.

> *Individual Consultants made comments suggesting that if I couldn't do the full quota of work, I should not be doing the work. It was suggested I was in the wrong specialty (bipolar disorder).*

This box shows suggestions by disabled doctors on what you can do to make it work.

Disabled doctors' recommendations for ways to help themselves

Being realistic

I feel that people with a disability have to accept that some roles may be inappropriate given the nature of their particular disability and the needs of the jobs in question.

We have to recognise when we are likely to have trouble doing something, and be honest enough to talk about it.

I need to allow more flexibility in meeting deadlines – i.e planning well ahead where possible to allow for "bad days" . Similarly I plan time off after I have been away at meetings abroad etc.

Showing commitment

They have been flexible with me, and with their support, I have not missed a deadline, or failed to produce whatever has been asked of me. In turn, I have been flexible with them as far as possible, e.g. if I am required to attend a meeting on a non-working day, I will make reasonable attempt to do so.

(Continued)

Being open

We can be helped by those of us with a disability being honest and open and acting as 'exemplars'.

I think a lot comes down to the abilities of the clinical teams surrounding the disabled doctor not to mollycoddle them. At the same time, we have to recognise when we are likely to have trouble doing something, and be honest enough to talk about it.

4.5 Gender still matters

As more women do science subjects in the final school years, women entrants to medicine have overtaken men in most countries. However, they are still in a minority in terms of senior posts and these proportional changes have still not filtered down to those very male surgical specialties. As well as a great lack of female role models, this is often because of negative role models who decided them firmly against surgery. There are also lifestyle decisions that make some women set their career aspirations differently to men. While they may be realistic about the difficulties of full-time work and a family, especially in hospital medicine (see Chapter 2), they also may not have good career guidance that would help them through some of the difficulties of 'having it all' that men seem to enjoy.

So women, don't change an old ambition because you feel a family life would be too difficult, not before you've really done your homework. If you've had a very bad experience with a role model in your once-chosen specialty, ask to try someone else rather than ruling out the whole specialty. And, if it feels impossible to train or work full time, get thorough human resource and deanery information and advice about other ways that you might train. *And,* if it still feels too difficult and you decide you need to 'settle for' something else, then enjoy it. You only have one life and sometimes only one go at enjoying your children, so following your heart is no bad thing: just make sure you get some career counselling first to find out just where your heart actually is!

4.6 Personality and career choice

Doctors want careers that are consistent with their personalities. Not surprising then, that your Myers Brigg Type, described in Chapter 2, is likely to be influential in a broad sense in how you choose your career. Remember that Type is only a preference, not an ability, and so you can always do the opposite of your type. Also, the MBTI has four dimensions and you are likely to find that, while some aspects of a job really energise you, others can have the opposite effect; for example, as an INFP GP you might love the relationships with your patients over time, but find keeping good data something of a grind. However, in terms of careers, you're going to have to do the job for a very long time, and that might sometimes feel uncomfortable if you choose everything opposite to how you'd most like to work.

Male UK doctors are more introverted than the general population and also more than female doctors. This is likely to make some hospital specialties more attractive than primary care since they can spend less time talking to patients and need not get to know them so well. This may be one reason that women are attracted to general practice. The same thing happens on the third dimension – the T–F that describes the way you prefer to make decisions. So male doctors prefer logical, rational methods (T), slightly more so than women doctors (and than patients), while women doctors, who are more strongly F, will usually base their decisions on values and will be more careful about the feelings of others. This may encourage them to spend longer with patients and colleagues (especially if they are extraverts) which will again encourage the choice of primary care. It may also steer them away from specialties where hard choices have to be made, around rationing, for example. Finally, it might partly explain why women are disciplined and complained about so much less frequently than men (see Chapter 12), not just because the Fs among them will show more tact, but also because they are more similar in type to their patients.

There is a variety of types in all jobs and in all specialties of medicine. However, it is inevitable that some types will favour particular roles. For example, laboratory-based doctors and other diagnosticians are predominantly ISTJs which is good because they don't need to mix too much with large groups of people, and they are very good at details and facts. Those in clinical specialties are predominantly INTJs – not so very different except on the data-gathering dimension where they contrast with the diagnosticians by being less concerned with detail and enjoying innovation and change more.

Remember that your Type is a combination of the four dimensions and so the 16 types will all behave differently and, although not inevitable, this will lead to somewhat different career paths. Because of this, it is important to get a more accurate identification of your type either professionally, or by using a book (see the bibliography) or on the net. Remember too that all Types are valuable and valued; they do not relate to your absolute skills, but to your preferences. Everyone can act at the other end of the dimension. For example, a friend of mine was President of his Royal College: a very people-intensive job that took him round the world interacting socially and professionally. Until he completed the MBTI and came out as an ISFJ with an off-the-scale score for Introversion, I would never have guessed he was introverted at all. Then I realised that he would from time to time vanish for a couple of days, shunning social contact on his small-holding, recovering from playing the extravert. But he played it well.

4.7 Choosing general practice or a hospital specialty

On the whole when they enter medical school, students report wanting prestigious careers (which they see primarily as surgery), but by final year they also care about the impact of different specialties on their personal lives and they then become more likely to go into general practice. However, different medical schools vary in the emphasis they give to 'scientific medicine' or to more community health issues, and this too influences the decision. There are also numerous individual reasons for choosing one rather than the other:

- Introverts are less likely to be happy in general practice.
- Doctors in primary care are going to need to be able to cope with greater uncertainty: they don't have all those tests and diagnosticians to hand and sometimes have to dare to wait and see. They have to sort out the common ailments from the rare disease. For many hospital specialties such as surgery the attractions are very different:

  People come in with a recognised spectrum of disease and you have a procedure which you do and if you do it properly they get better. It's immediate results, quick turnover and lots of research. It's easy to get a sense of achievement.

- GPs are more likely to put lifestyle issues first: wanting a family, a dog, a walk on a Sunday, a pub where they know people:

  I can make my work more flexible and I actually have some kind of life outside medicine.

  [In order to help me decide] I looked to see if the registrars were happy with their jobs. That convinced me to be a GP!

> Paul knew that he didn't want to be a surgeon but wasn't exactly sure what he did want to do. He enjoyed meeting people and dealing with a wide range of ages and types of patients. He was tempted by general (internal) medicine, paediatrics or becoming a GP. However he also needed to plan his life around his wife's career in intensive care anaesthesiology. She had limited geographical options for her training and worked complex rotas. Paul decided the best thing to do was apply for GP training as that would offer him (and them) the greatest flexibility.

- Those in primary care have to enjoy seeing their patients over time: year-in, year-out. They need to like the elderly and the young and deal with illnesses that can't be cured. All this continuity is enormously attractive for some people and completely repugnant to others, perhaps because of differing attachment styles:

  I don't like old people and I don't like children and I can't stand trivial illnesses and people whining (trainee surgeon).

- People with secure styles of attachment have been found more likely to go into primary care roles. The four attachment styles, arising from our earliest relationships, are: *secure*, measured by agreement with statements such as 'It is easy for me to get emotionally close to others', and 'I am comfortable depending on people'; *self-reliant*, answering yes to statements like 'I prefer not to have other people depend on me'; *cautious* – 'I am somewhat uncomfortable being close to others'; and *support-seeking* – 'I worry about having others not accept me'.
- GPs are largely high in their desire for professional freedom, so running their own businesses to a large degree suits them well. However, these arrangements are changing in the UK with the arrival of primary care businesses which employ doctors, so GPs may become managed just as hospital doctors are.

Some of these reasons for choosing general practice will be equally applicable to why you might choose psychiatry.

4.8 Discover your career anchor

The American psychologist Edgar Schein has proposed that you need to discover the particular element of medicine that is essential to keep you satisfied at work. This might be intellectual challenge, working in a team, talking to patients or doing practical procedures. You might need to do regular teaching or research. Without this anchor in your professional life you will feel frustrated, so if you love clinical work don't become a full-time medical manager and vice versa. Finding your anchor means reflecting carefully on what gives you most satisfaction at work. Write down what excites you, the events and activities that give you most pleasure, the things you look forward to doing each day or each week. Keep a diary of your daily routine and mark against the different components of the day and how you feel about them.

Schein describes a series of common anchors – technical competence (e.g. surgery or radiology), managerial competence (clinical director), creativity (GP business partner), security (rheumatologist) or autonomy (researcher). You need to discover what gives you the most 'buzz' out of being a doctor and plan that element clearly into your career pathway for at least part of the time. That way you won't become frustrated and disillusioned by missing out on what you like best about medicine.

4.9 So how do you choose?

You will gather that there are no hard and fast rules for this, but certainly some ideas on how to get started.

- Do a Myers Brigg assessment and think about how different roles will fit with your personality type.
- Be realistic about your abilities. Ask your friends, colleagues and trainers.
- Think about what you enjoy most and what you do best; for example, interacting with people, achieving technical skills, managerial tasks, excitement and risk and teaching. Ask yourself to what extent you enjoy autonomy and what role is likely to provide it in the amount you might like. No role will give you everything you want, but you should try to match those you enjoy the most.
- Think about how well you cope with uncertainty. If you are an S (rather than an N) this may make some jobs, such as general practice, more difficult for you to enjoy.
- Try to get brief 'tasters' of the specialties that attract you. Don't be put off by one experience of a poor role model.
- Get support and careers advice from your educational supervisors or from a careers counsellor. If you feel you want to change career paths you should get more professional advice that really looks at you and any obstacles stopping your job satisfaction, since it is now becoming more difficult to switch direction.

Bibliography

Ciechanowski PS, Russo JE, Katon WJ, Walker EA. Attachment theory in health care: the influence of relationship style on medical students' specialty choice. *Med Educ* 2004;**38**:262–70.

Firth-Cozens J. Improving the health of psychiatrists. *Adv Psychiatr Treat* 2007;**13**:161–8.

Firth-Cozens J, Caceres Lema V, Firth RA. Specialty choice, stress and personality: their relationships over time. *Hosp Med* 1999;**60**:751–5.

Hughes PH, Baldwin DC, Sheehan DV, et al. Resident physician substance use by specialty, *Am J Psychiatr* 1992;**149**:1348–54.

Hummerow JM (ed.). *New Directions in Career Planning and the Workplace. Practical Strategies for Counsellors.* 1991, CPP Books, Palo Alto.

Petchey, et al. 'Ending up a GP': a qualitative study of junior doctors' perceptions of general practice as a career. *Fam Pract* 1997;**14**:194–8.

Schein, EH. *Career Anchors: Self Assessment.* 2006, Pfeiffer, San Francisco.

Chapter 5 **Dealing with stress**

Stress, depression, trauma – we realise they're not the most positive way to start a chapter and already you may have decided you simply don't want to know! But you've read the statistics about the problems that affect a good proportion of doctors and you've seen that you do have objectively difficult jobs throughout your careers. When you list some of the stressors – breaking bad news, making life-threatening errors, cutting people, carrying out intimate examinations, causing pain, dealing with difficult people, conflicts in your personal life – it's hardly surprising that the pressures of your job are sometimes going to make your stress levels zoom above normal. Most of the time it will be only a temporary rise, and a good sleep and some warm company will bring your levels back to normal. Not surprisingly, the longer they are elevated, the more entrenched the symptoms will become, and so the harder they will be to change. This is particularly the case when the problems are not just work related, but happening at home as well.

5.1 Recognise it!

The very first thing to do is diagnose yourself: the sooner you recognise the problem could be stress, the sooner you can do something about it. Just to remind you, the next box shows some of the symptoms of stress.

You know better than anyone that many of these symptoms may indicate a physical cause rather than a psychological one, but it is still important to bear in mind some of the things that have been happening to you lately and whether they could be causing you to feel different, perhaps to change your behaviour. If you have doubts about this, ask friends whether they have noticed any differences in how you seem to them. Similarly, if a friend or colleague seems different to you nowadays, is perhaps less easy to get on with, or isn't mixing like he or she used to do, then don't be slow in asking if anything is wrong.

How to Survive in Medicine. By © Jenny Firth-Cozens. Published 2010 Blackwell Publishing.

Physical	**Behavioural**	**Emotional**
Palpitations	More irritable, angry	Worrying a lot
Chest pain	Absence from work	Checking things more
Cold sweats	Overwork	Feeling irritable or tense
Dizziness	Avoiding people or situations	Depressed
Headaches	Insomnia	Confidence dropping
Backache	Concentration problems	Agitated
Nausea	Less interest in sex	Feelings of dread
Butterflies in your stomach		Feelings of rage
Muscle tension		Eating more or less
Exhaustion		Drinking and smoking more

Because chronic stress underlies a lot of other problems, it's important to understand how it happens and how we should be tackling it. One way to understand stress is set out in Figure 5.1 adapted from a model by Professor Tom Cox. This proposes that it is a combination of reality – the job is objectively difficult – and perceptions: what is judged as a problem and how stressful that problem is will still differ for different people. The model sees stress as a mismatch between our abilities and the demands placed on us, but also between what we *see* as our capabilities and resources and what we *see* as the demands and difficulties.

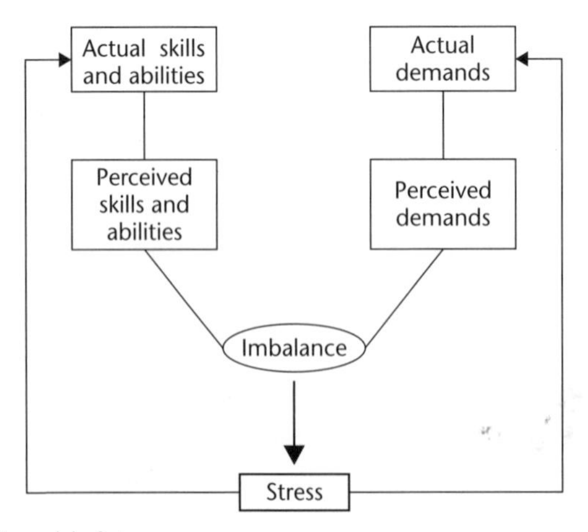

Figure 5.1 A model of stress.

There are various ways this mismatch can occur: our actual capabilities and actual demands may not be the same as our perceived ones. For example, I might see myself as not having the skills to tackle this new job, and I'm starting to worry about it seriously: will I fail to please my boss or impress my colleagues, will I make a mistake that will cost me dear, will we still be able to pay the mortgage if I lose this post, will she or he still love me – and so on. Frightening, catastrophising thoughts! If we look at the figure we can see that my stress emerges because I see the demands as greater than my skills to meet them. But this is where I need to check up on the accuracy of my perceptions.

The first thing to do with this model is to test out the 'actual' demands: what is *actually* expected of you. If you're worrying that someone might be thinking you're performing badly or not as well as you could, then check it out with them. This is usually done by consulting those who set the demands: checking on protocols, talking with your boss or your partner to get them to be precise about what they are expecting of you and how you will both know that this is being achieved. You are unlikely to hear anything worse than you're fearing already, and usually you'll hear a whole lot better. But if things are as bad or worse than you think, then at least you know now and you can begin to do something about it. If the person you consult uses vague words like 'take more responsibility' or 'spend less time with patients', get them to be precise so you know what the demand actually involves: 'How will we know I'm being more responsible?' 'How many patients should I see? Will this include psychiatric problems as well as physical?' Young doctors in particular, but also new consultants, need more guidance on what must be done, what can be left and what is urgent.

Remember that everyone has different skills and different strengths, so we are all relatively unskilled in some areas. Moreover, research has shown the more we lack a skill, the less insight we have about that: as our skills increase, our estimation of those skills actually goes down at first as it becomes more accurate. So if you find you do need more skills, realise that is normal – no one is perfect – and find out how to get them.

5.2 Taking control and letting it go

Sometimes you can be your own worst enemy: a high achiever at school and university, perhaps talented at sport or music, or both, you set yourself high standards in all you do. You see yourself as a problem-solver – at work, in the home, and with family and friends. Faced with a clinical challenge, maybe you rise to the occasion to 'sort it out'. You are often the one others depend on, and perhaps you get frustrated when things don't work out successfully 100% of the time.

Yet all too often in the world of health care, problems don't have easy or possible solutions. Patients get intractable pain, don't respond to antibiotics, fail to survive major surgery. Despite all you do, patients die on you. Some fail to take your advice. Others make formal complaints about the care you offer, despite all you've tried to do for them. The managers don't seem to understand what needs to be done, or the pressure that you are under. And society too has great expectations of you, as you do of yourself. Yet you are not super-human. You can't solve everyone's problems. One key thing to sort out is 'what is possible?' in each situation – what it is possible to solve, and what is beyond even your expertise. Learning that sort of wisdom is a positive way forward, both for now and for the future. Endlessly trying to solve a problem where there is no easy solution, or where the solution is beyond your control, will mostly likely lead to stress. This might be the diabetic patient who refuses to take regular blood checks, the drug misuser who fails repeatedly in their promises to give up the habit or the asthmatics who overuse their inhalers. You feel responsible and get more and more irritated and frustrated. Yet ultimately you need to recognise it is the patient's decision, as long as they have been properly informed by you of the issues and choices they face.

With health care systems across the world facing increasing regulation and greater financial pressures, you may feel threatened that your ability to make clinical decisions is being affected by external factors such as protocols and cost-saving measures beyond your control. Feeling that your participation in decision-making is being reduced is a real stressor: we all like to feel in control over the way we achieve an agreed outcome. Maybe you might instead do this best by getting involved politically or nationally in the profession, or locally with management. Otherwise, you need to find areas of your work or your life outside work where you can participate fully and feel in control of the way things happen.

Once you've got a more accurate picture of the thing that is causing you a problem, then you need to ask the crucial question: is it controllable or not?

John was a high profile palliative care specialist with a key role working in the community and in a local hospice. He had campaigned successfully to raise money for the hospice building and sustained a key teaching and research commitment. Then the local primary care trust took over the management of the hospice services, effectively removing leadership from the clinicians, and multiple problems ensued. John became perplexed and confused by this, attempting to sort things out as he had previously done. But his efforts got nowhere. He became increasingly stressed and depressed. It was only when he began to talk things through with a mentor that he began to understand the dynamics of what had happened, and could then begin to disengage from the stressors, focussing on what he could realistically achieve, both within his work and elsewhere.

It's always worth having a few goes to test out how controllable something is; whether it's a wall made of brick or one made of paper that you can break through the moment you start to push.

What you can do in terms of gaining control will be partly to do with the job and partly to do with changing yourself. You might, for example, find that you can do more or deal with the job more easily if you look after yourself better physically: that you cut down on alcohol, stop smoking, get some exercise and eat healthily. You may be thinking grandmothers and eggs at this point, but are you really doing all this? Keep a diary and find out. Once you have an accurate picture of the demands that are expected, and you've got yourself sufficiently strong to meet them but you still find they are more than you can do, then it may be necessary to get help to organise things differently in your work or outside of it, or look around to see where extra support can be found.

However, if it seems as though the wall is immovable, certainly at the moment, then you have to let it go: stop wasting energy struggling with it and worrying about it and instead spend your energies on helping yourself to stay relaxed and cheerful and true to yourself despite the problem. This is only a version of what happens when you're agitating in a traffic jam, willing the cars to move, and you suddenly realise you can do nothing about it and the traffic will start moving when it does. And when you realise that, you feel so much better. If there still seem to be no available solutions at the moment, then you need to accept that the problem as it stands is currently uncontrollable. The next step is to break down the elements that make up the problem and begin to tackle whichever ones you can. Don't struggle on your own: using colleagues or friends to help you do this can help enormously, even if they know nothing about being a doctor. But also remember that everything changes in time, so nudge that wall occasionally to see if it's still so unmovable and, in the mean time, look after yourself.

5.3 The eye of the beholder

One reason it's good to talk things out with others is that different people react differently to the same situation (see Chapter 2). Research from the 1980s, when unemployment was very high, showed that most of the unemployed found this a stressful and depressing experience: in terms of the model above, their skills and capabilities outstripped the demands. However, a small group coped very well with the situation, viewing the whole experience as an opportunity for doing things they'd always wanted to do. Some spent long hours each day developing an early yearning to paint or write; others became politically active, or put enormous energy into a particular charity. They could make the most of the situation because they perceived it differently, for all sorts of reasons. Perhaps they were optimists: this seems a personality characteristic that's good for physical and mental health (even if pessimists are sometimes more accurate in their predictions). Perhaps they had grown up in a family where members were encouraged to follow hobbies they enjoyed, or one that encouraged their self-esteem, or let them believe many things were possible for them. Perhaps they had simply learnt that they were only happy when they were actively doing something, or when they were with others, and this knowledge helped them choose some activity that would be beneficial.

Once they've been tested, the perceptions boxes in the diagram might reveal themselves as very different to the reality boxes. If this seems to happen to you a lot, then we need to think why. Many of the reasons are to do with our personalities, background experience or life events. For example, if I consistently see my skills as less than they really are, perhaps I had a parent who never seemed satisfied however much I achieved; perhaps a recent life event, like the end of a relationship or a bullying boss, has sapped my confidence; or maybe losing a parent early on made me feel responsible when things go wrong. These are individual reasons that can make us sometimes think in particular ways and so underestimate our abilities. Gaining insight into them can sometimes be enough to begin changing successfully.

5.4 Keeping a diary

It's often useful to keep a diary to log when you feel stressed: what seems to precipitate it, what else is happening at the time and what helps it; for example, which thoughts you can use to challenge the negative ones. You're looking to see if any pattern or insight emerges in terms of what seems to bring on the feelings, and what seems to alleviate them. For example, I might find that all authority figures seem to cause me discomfort and make me feel they are criticising me, but challenging myself over this might let me recognise that I've still got good references so they apparently thought reasonably well of me. Gaining insight into these background reasons for the way we think is helpful, though difficult to do alone and not always necessary. If you find that you have no idea why you seem to be always overwhelmed with tasks that others tackle easily, or why you find most bosses or managers impossible, then diaries can still help you to find ways to intervene. Do you feel worse if you drink the night before; does walking or cycling to work make you feel better than taking public transport; does talking to a friend regularly get the day into perspective for both of you?

Diaries also help you to challenge your perceptions; for example by focussing on others instead of yourself. Does your senior colleague *always* seem unfriendly, or is it just on Mondays? Could he or she have had a bad time at home? Are they actually not feeling well? Do they look tired? Writing down other reasons for what we see as the cause of our stress can help.

5.5 Feeling overwhelmed

Some people really love finishing things (Js in Myers Brigg terms), but medicine could be seen as a job that can never be finished. There will always be something else to do. We discuss demands much more in Chapter 10 but one useful reminder now is that, rather than feel that you are under an unending river of demands that is swamping you and that you struggle and struggle to get to the end of, accept that there is no end – this is the job – and instead begin to think in terms of priorities and how to finish those. That will give you a sense of achievement and you will know that the most important things are getting done. If you are left with a large pile of less important things, you may find that someone else can do them better

> Margaret is a trainee anaesthetist, divorced with two young children under four. Her ex-husband has just made consultant in another part of the country, and the children rarely see him. She has managed to get a flexible training post but feels this will hold her back from real success and make people think her second-rate in some way so that her career will suffer. By keeping diaries, challenging her perceptions both herself and by talking to others, and joining together a group of women in a similar situation, she found she could cope much better. She realised she spent a lot of time furious with her ex-husband, not just for letting her and her children down, but because he had done well in terms of his ambitions and she felt this had been because of her sacrifice. She wanted him to fail at something. She was sad but relieved when she admitted that she could do nothing about him, other than to make sure she was reasonably provided for: that he was outside her control. She also realised that she felt guilty about the children having so little of her, and guilty about her work and whether people felt she didn't pull her weight. By checking with her seniors that her work was sufficiently high quality and finding that they admired how well she ran a difficult agenda, she was able to let that go and appreciate that she would only have three more difficult years; that she had the pleasure of the children and would start to enjoy them properly rather than resent her ex-husband's freedom; and that she would easily catch up with her ambitions in what was really not too long. She found the children responded well to the extra attention from a less irritable mother, and they all gained more pleasure from each other. She started a self-help group with a few women colleagues, ostensibly calling it a book group, and found it invaluable in terms of being able to express what she felt at times, using each other for support, and just having a laugh.

and so start to delegate. If you're still too junior to do that, then make sure you maintain good relationships with others on the ward or in the practice. Nurses will usually be very willing to help a doctor who is consistently pleasant to them, who takes time to notice how they are feeling and who includes them in decision-making.

Tackle your stress by addressing any of the four boxes in the model in a variety of ways so that you balance demands and capabilities more equally.

There are two other areas, highly related to stress, which are rarely discussed in terms of doctors' health, but which should be: anxiety and post-traumatic stress disorder (PTSD).

5.6 Don't panic!

Anxiety has only rarely been measured in doctors, but where it has been it was found to be high. For example, a study of GPs found 19% showed clinical evidence of anxiety, especially if they lived alone and had high levels of on-call duties, and another 22% were borderline for anxiety. There were no gender differences. Further evidence for high levels of anxiety comes from the studies that show benzodiazapines to be one of the drugs most commonly used by doctors – often self-prescribed and dreadfully addictive. Occasional short bouts of anxiety and panic in your jobs are not unusual – most of your colleagues will have experienced just the same, but not talked about it. But taking drugs is not the answer to a situation which is long-lasting: your career. You need to find other well-tested answers.

As you know, anxiety has most of the same symptoms as stress, but writ large and much more fearful. In case you've never had one, a panic attack feels like every stress symptom coming at once, often triggered by a fearful thought or situation that leads to hyperventilation. Tackle your breathing by learning to slow it through relaxation and you'll probably not have one again; do nothing and you may find they develop into a cycle of episodes which involve, not the original thought, but a fear of fear itself.

Some doctors, particularly but not always the younger ones, use alcohol and other drugs to quell the anxiety and stress they feel. These might appear to work quite well in the short run, but are disastrous when they become the main means of tackling the inevitable daily stressors in the job or at home, as will be discussed in Chapter 9. Much better to learn relaxation or yoga and to use it to tackle the stressors and to slow your breathing. However, if you find your anxiety or panic attacks are not controllable by you without these drugs, then get help for the problem. Suffering in this way is depressing and unnecessary. Cognitive behaviour therapy is extremely effective in this area and all clinical psychologists and many psychiatrists and counsellors will be able to provide it.

5.7 Sometimes work is traumatic

The other area that is under-researched in doctors is PTSD. We know that police and ambulance personnel suffer PTSD in significant numbers from dealing with the human aftermath of accidents and fires and murders, but we know little about the effects on doctors. Just to remind you, the symptoms of PTSD involve:

- Flash-backs of the trauma and painful emotions in thinking about it;
- Avoidance of people or of things or places that might trigger memories, increased use of alcohol or other drugs to blot out thinking about it;
- Numbness of feelings;
- Very short temper, feeling irritable or angry;
- Disrupted sleep or nightmares;
- Difficulty concentrating and poor work performance.

In a study following health workers involved in treating victims of the Omagh bombing, the individual factors that caused long-term problems were: having previous emotional problems, previous similar traumas or trying to cope by not thinking about it. Their alcohol use had increased. Those who did best in the months after the event had discussed it openly with friends or counsellors and had cut down on their alcohol use rather than increasing it.

5.8 Coming from overseas

Overseas doctors have particular problems that others don't experience. They often arrive without a real sense of the country, the customs and the background as well as practical knowledge that makes life easier: how to find somewhere to live, open a bank account, register with a GP, deal with electricity companies and the Inland Revenue. It can be overwhelming and lonely. Women in particular seem to suffer, and their suicide rate has been found to be high. If you are from overseas, use all the support on offer and try to find more, so that you investigate local evening classes as well as any special ones offered by your postgraduate deaneries or other training establishments. Although it's tempting and important to mix with people from your country, make sure you also join local groups where you can so that communication skills improve and you can ask local people what to do in situations that are new.

5.9 Financial issues

Turbulence in the world's financial markets reminds us that money, especially the lack of it, contributes greatly to stress and anxiety. Doctors should be relatively immune to such concerns, as most eventually have good salaries and a safe job. However, things can be very difficult in the first few years as many of you will graduate with huge debts just at a time when you might want to do the ordinary things in life like buying a house and raising a family. If you feel that this is very tricky to manage, then that is fair enough – it's a problem to be managed while you wait a bit longer to have the sort of remuneration that you expected.

But if you find yourself getting furious about something you feel you can do little about – that is, earn more now – then you need to apply some of the lessons in this and later chapters to address how you think about the situation. It's worth realising, for example, that you can always leave medicine. This would be a pity after so much study and such a good potential life still to come, but it is an option. Knowing you have a choice is often very helpful as it then becomes your decision to stay and hopefully to enjoy the route you've chosen. Some of you may feel you deserve to start spending – but this can lead to further problems in the future, so hang on until you've really learnt what everyday living costs. One approach is to write down what you actually spend for a whole week, and see what that tells you about yourself: where can you cut back and what 'treat' is a necessity.

But even when your salary has risen, this may not be enough to prevent you from being anxious about money, or from needing more cash. This is because individuals vary greatly in how they manage their financial affairs. You may be a cautious or a reckless spender. You may or may not like to save for a rainy day. Going over your finances with someone else – your partner, a friend, an accountant or a financial advisor – might help you see where you can manage better.

Often the bigger picture is the key – what are your expectations for the future? If you imagine you will have a large house, a second home in the country, expensive cars and a lavish lifestyle, then either you need to think again or plan a medical career with a lucrative private practice. If, however, the need to earn all the money to maintain such a way of life starts to burn you out, then perhaps a wiser response would be to trim back and re-calibrate your expectations. The solutions are in your hands to a greater degree than is sometimes realised.

5.10 Coping well

There is no doubt that, whether it's stress, anxiety or PTSD, the worst way to cope is to try to dismiss or deny it and bottle up the feelings you might have had. In a comparison of young doctors who had been above threshold for stress on two occasions over two years with those below threshold on both occasions, the main differences in their strategies for coping with stress were that the 'never stressed' asked for help more often and the 'always stressed' tried more often to dismiss the event.

Acknowledging your stress and talking about it to someone helps not only your mental health but also your physical health. A paper in the *Journal of the American Medical Association,* following a long line of research on the positive effects of discussing traumas, found that the symptoms of rheumatoid arthritis and of eczema reduced significantly in those who described a trauma compared to those who described an insignificant event. Other studies have found beneficial effects in terms of the immune system of speaking about trauma and, to a lesser extent, of writing about it. Whatever else you do, don't bottle it up!

5.11 Summary

1 **Recognise what's happening**
In all these situations – whether you're stressed, anxious or suffering from PTSD – the most important first step in stopping the symptoms is to recognise that you have them. Denial or avoidance of stressors has time and again been shown to be the worst possible strategy for dealing with problems, whether simple stress or PTSD. And avoiding issues by using alcohol or drugs will make the whole thing 10 times worse. Talk to someone close who you won't see as simply critical, or be a scientist and keep a diary to help you see better what is happening; for example, recognising the possibility that:
   - your irritability may not all be to do with dealing with difficult patients or an unappreciative boss;
   - despite your long hours, what you have been doing shouldn't really make you this exhausted;
   - your drinking or smoking have definitely increased lately;
   - friends or family are telling you that you have a problem.

2 **Change your capabilities and resources**
   - Get healthy: improve your diet, increase your enjoyable exercise, take some early nights, decrease alcohol, coffee and cigarettes.
   - Learn to relax or meditate: join a yoga class or buy yourself a relaxation tape. It's a physical skill, so practise it daily or it won't work!
   - Take up a pasttime that uses quite different skills to those you use in the workplace – something that will take you somewhere else, like music or cooking or painting or a sport.
   - Ask for help in the workplace and outside. Don't wait till it's offered: it might not be.

3 Deal with the demands and pressures on you
- Write down your priorities and space them out more sensibly wherever you can. Discuss this with your tutor, boss or colleague.
- Ask for help: two pairs of hands and two minds are almost always better than one. Nurses can be very helpful indeed if you ask them.
- Don't programme your leisure time: don't think up a list of tasks to do around the home, and don't party till all hours. Rest and socialise with people you care about.

4 Change your perceptions
- Learn to recognise negative thoughts about your capabilities and challenge them.
- Write down a list of your successes, small as well as large.
- Ask for guidance of what's expected of you, and ask for feedback now on whether or not you are achieving it.
- Check that you're not setting yourself too high goals so the demands are always massive and success is unlikely.
- Realise that you can't control everything in life.
- Accept what can't be changed.

Bibliography

Atik Y. Personal coaching for senior doctors. BMJ Career focus; 8 April 2000; 2–3.

Cozens J. *Nervous Breakdown: What Is It? What Causes It? Who Can Help?* 1993, Piatkus, London.

Davis M. Intern discussion group: a supportive educational experience for junior doctors. *Hosp Med* 1999;**60**:435–9.

Davis M, Eshelman ER. *The Relaxation and Stress Reduction Workbook*. 2008, New Harbinger Publications, Oakland, CA.

Elkin A. *Stress Management for Dummies*. 1999, John Wiley & Sons, Chichester.

Kabat-Zinn J. *Wherever You Go, There You Are*. 2004, Piatkus, London.

Rich AJ. An induction programme for first-appointment overseas doctors. *Med Teach* 1998;**20**:473–5.

Slowther A, et al. *Non UK Qualified Doctors and Good Medical Practice: The Experience of Working Within a Different Professional Framework*. Report for the General Medical Council, 2009.

Tattersall AJ, Bennett P, Pugh S. Stress and coping in hospital doctors. *Stress Med* 1999;**15**:109–113.

Chapter 6 **Down in the dumps**

Down in the dumps, in the doldrums, despondent, dejected, desperate: why do so many adjectives describing depression always seem to start with D? There are so many English words for feeling down that it's clearly a very common part of our human condition. Most of us feel depressed at some time or another, and a quarter of us will have a clinical depression at some point in our lives, perhaps with obvious reason, perhaps with none that we can recognise.

Reported estimates for the levels of depression in doctors vary widely, though they are always equal to or above the community norms. This variation occurs not only because different studies use different instruments, but also because doctors are more likely to become depressed at different points in their career than others, and in different working environments. In this sense depression is likely at least in part to be due to the job rather than only to what we carry with us in terms of genetics, early experience and life events. This chapter will look at the individual and job-related causes of depression, and ways to tackle them.

6.1 Recognising depression

Depression can arrive suddenly, within days or weeks, or it can be so gradual that it seems to be a normal part of someone's life. It is often experienced alongside anxiety, while alcohol and drug abuse will often mask it both to the depressed doctor and to those around him or her. While it should be one of the easiest conditions to recognise in yourself, for some reason, unless very acute, it isn't always so obvious. The clinical symptoms are set out in every book of psychiatry:

Tearful	A sense of foreboding
Feeling tired	Lower libido
A marked loss of pleasure	Feeling hopeless
Losing your appetite	Hard to make decisions
Early waking	Problems remembering things
Lowered self-esteem	Thoughts of suicide

Nevertheless, intelligent people seem to find all sorts of ways to ignore these symptoms. In doctors this can sometimes be due to the features of their work – because of the hours and conditions and content of the job you might regularly experience a daily loss of pleasure, early waking, less desire for sex, tiredness, and a sense of foreboding that you've not done every you should every minute of the day. Doctors can often fail to recognise that they are depressed because they are so used to these job-related effects.

Anger too can be used to mask sadness. People say: 'I don't dare to stop feeling angry because I'm scared of what's under it.' Doctors often cover their depression with overwork: busy, busy, busy; walking fast, talking fast, producing papers, reorganising the clinic, getting grants – and then surprising everyone by crashing into recognisably deep depression or even suicide. Depression is a dangerous disease for a doctor. Like farmers, they have at their fingertips far too many ways to attempt suicide and the knowledge to make it successful. Not surprising that they are amongst the highest risk groups for taking their own lives. The most dangerous times are in their first postgraduate year and their first year as consultant, and the most dangerous specialty groups are anaesthesiologists, community health doctors, GPs and psychiatrists.

Cliff struggled with depressive feeling for many years. He reached a stage in mid-career where his low energy levels, poor sleep and inability to concentrate were beginning to affect the care of his patients. As a GP himself, he realised that he needed help, but worried about what he saw as the stigma of being diagnosed with clinical depression. At last he visited his own GP who referred him to the local clinical psychology service for cognitive behaviour therapy, and recommended a course of SSRI anti-depressant tablets. The GP also offered time off work to give the tablets a chance to work. Cliff struggled with all this but, having talked things through with a close friend, he agreed to take his doctor's advice. Once in therapy, he found that the chance to talk about some things openly for the first time gave him a new perspective on issues affecting his current life.

Other symptoms, especially for men, involve a longing to 'escape' – their jobs, their relationships, perhaps their lives. This seems more common in the mid-life period when they sometimes get a first glimpse of their futures and their mortality. And men too will often show their depression through bad behaviour of some sort. In a longitudinal study of depressed 18 year olds, their records from when they were young children showed that while the little girls were very good and strict with themselves, the boys were even then remarkable for behaving badly. For anyone facing discipline for bad behaviour, it is worth thinking first if the underlying cause might be depression.

6.2 Causes and cures

Chronic stress and stressful life events can slip into depression by affecting the stress hormones and through the negative beliefs that often go alongside: we are adapted to think the worst given even a hint that things are going wrong. This allowed us to make our escape more quickly; for example, 'That noise is a bear and I'll get eaten'. The current thoughts – such as 'I'm to blame' or 'I'm not good enough' or 'I can't manage' – become depression-inducing in themselves and so we can easily get into a vicious circle of stressful events, negative thoughts and depression. Anxiety too frequently goes hand in hand with depression through a similar mechanism, and people will often experience depressive symptoms when they suffer from PTSD. In both cases the symptoms of anxiety or PTSD will make them wonder if they are going mad or, if panic is involved, that they are dying. These thoughts and those that follow on may, not surprisingly, trigger depression. For this reason, learn how to recognise early signs of stress in yourself, and treat it in any of the ways that work for you (Chapter 5).

A lack of social support has been linked to depression for many years, especially if you're missing someone in whom you can confide and who confides in you. When you are working hard with long or unsociable hours, it is very easy to let friendships go and socialising turn meaningless. As health care becomes more intensive, modelled increasingly on a factory, the ward teams, medical firms and general practices that were relatively unchanging for decades have now become a thing of the past, and the team support that they offered has often vanished alongside. This means that the workplace is less and less the arena in which you will get the right level of friendly interaction and so you will increasingly need to make sure you have some sort of social support outside of work.

The type of social life you need will depend on the type of person you are. Extraverts (Es) will be happy with having a reasonably large circle of friends and confiding in them easily: this is the way they relieve their stress. However, they can become very lonely very quickly if they are without these interactions and so they need to be particularly vigilant in developing new contacts if they have recently moved jobs or houses. Introverts (Is), on the other hand, will prefer a small number of friends they can depend upon but will prefer to treat their stress by withdrawing. They are less likely to discuss their problems unless they have a reliable and trustworthy one-to-one relationship, perhaps with a partner. As it is so important to have that sort of support, both extraverts and introverts need to ensure they have at least one person that they can open their hearts to and who will also be open with them.

In a study of the stressors experienced by intensivists, those who were *not* depressed said the things that caused them the most stress were the difficulty of allocating a bed when the intensive care unit was full, and being over-stretched at times: both job-related factors. On the other hand, those who *were* depressed gave factors to do with relationships: the effects of stress on their personal life and the lack of recognition of their contribution by others. Relationships matter for all of us, but when you are depressed, they often matter more and they are usually viewed more negatively. Carving out time to make sure you can enjoy a personal or family life is crucial, even if it's less than you would like. In terms of the lack of recognition or appreciation, you need to see that the cause of this is that everyone is so busy that appreciation often slips out the window. If you have a partner or someone at work that you can talk to, make sure you check with them periodically that the work you do is up to scratch and even ask them what they appreciate you for and what you could do better. This way you can get used to getting feedback – both positive and negative – and get support in changing where necessary. And if you are part of a team, start showing your appreciation to others and they might just learn to do the same to you!

Self-criticism and self-blame are raised when you are depressed. However, as we showed in Chapter 2, they can also be a personality trait or a learnt way of thinking which may not involve depression but which can trigger it when job stress or life events happen. When something unexpected occurs – something good or bad – we tend to provide causes or attributional thoughts for it and these attributions lead to particular emotions and particular actions. So if we are walking in a wood and we get a sharp blow to the back of our head, we might think 'It's a mugger', in which case we will feel fear and run. If we think 'It's an irritating boy throwing conkers' we will feel angry and turn to confront him. And if we think 'The wind has got up and is breaking twigs off the trees', we will rub our heads and walk on.

Why we think one thing and not another is partly due to our previous experiences and partly to our personality, and also even to how we're feeling today. However, some attributions for negative events are more likely to make us feel depressed than others: those which are internal (blaming ourselves), stable (will last for a long time, like personality), general (affect everything) and uncontrollable (nothing we can do to change them) are the most likely to predict depression. Those who are neither self-critical nor prone to blame only external forces might decide it's the hospital system that is mainly responsible, but also realise their part in it, while seeing this as a one-off difficulty that doesn't affect most of their care and which can be eradicated by getting extra training, writing clearer notes and so on. They are also more likely to take credit for themselves when they do something well. Someone with consistently low self-criticism is more likely to provide external causes when things go wrong, and less likely to do so when things are good.

Someone who is consistently self-critical will do the opposite. This way of thinking is particularly risky in medicine because, let's face it, things go wrong quite often, sometimes with potentially devastating consequences. In situations like that, when errors or less than perfect care takes place, a self-critical doctors will say: 'I failed; it was all my fault; I should have done X, Y, Z; I'll never make a good doctor; it's the same with everything I do'. Etcetera, etcetera. Although they may try to think the opposite and see all responsibility resting elsewhere (on the pathology laboratory or X-ray for being so slow, or the nurses for not telling them something, or a colleague for being absent, or the patient for being unreasonable and so on), blaming others brings no relief to someone who is by temperament self-critical. In addition, it means they don't learn from what goes wrong, and it can make them less than popular with colleagues. When things go well, self-critical people are usually slow in acknowledging their success, so they are poor at giving themselves strokes or gold stars.

What you need to do is to allocate responsibility reasonably so that you can see both the external and individual factors that lead to a positive or negative event. It's never helpful to give a cause for a negative event that suggests you have some permanent characteristic which will always affect things badly in the future and which is uncontrollable; for example:

- that you lack intelligence, as opposed to needing certain skills which can be learnt;
- that nobody seems to like you, as opposed to that specific person might not like you but those others clearly do, and anyway, you don't expect everyone at work to like you and vice versa;
- that you are an inadequate or worthless person, rather than one who, when you add them up, does a host of valuable tasks each day.

As we described above, the causes or attributions you make lead to very different emotions and then to different consequences, so those causal thoughts matter and you might need to challenge and change them regularly to help change your mood. If you find this too difficult to do yourself, then approaching a psychologist or a counsellor who has cognitive-behavioural training will help to get your started.

Perfectionism is related to self-criticism and that too can lead to depression, especially in medicine where perfect care is rarely possible and what is 'good enough' can be difficult to evaluate. Both self-criticism and perfectionism are temperaments which are also likely to make you need appreciation – someone other than you to tell you you've done well. However, although most patients are still quite appreciative, praise and gratitude are sadly rarely expressed by colleagues. A few strokes by team members will never go amiss.

Needless to say, appraisal and accreditation can be major stressors for someone who is a perfectionist or who is particularly self-critical, certainly if the person doing the appraising doesn't have enough training or doesn't appreciate quite how much this means to you.

Sona always feared that she never quite knew enough medicine and that her ignorance would be found out. Throughout medical school and GP training she worried about each assessment and assignment, even though her grades were high and she ended up with a distinction in her Membership exam. Faced with preparing for her annual appraisal, and knowing that this would contribute to her five-yearly revalidation folder, she had become increasingly anxious and upset. Her appraiser (a GP from a local practice) failed to grasp Sona's concerns and also seemed unsure of the fine detail of the appraisal process. This further unnerved Sona, who became frightened that, not only was she going to fall short of the standards set for revalidation, but that the process itself would be derailed by the incompetence (as she saw it) of the appraiser.

Sona was able to give feedback on her appraisal experience to the local GP tutor, who signalled to the local primary care trust (PCT) that all was not well. The PCT arranged for a review of the process, reassuring Sona and appointing a different, more experienced appraiser for the coming year. This appraisal proved much more successful and gave Sona renewed self-confidence.

Loss in all its forms is a major cause of depression. Of course, many of the life events that affect us are forms of loss – not just that we lose people we are close to, but loss of jobs, health, mobility, support, for example – and that is an important reason for the effects that the events have upon us. If you have lost a parent when you are a young person, you might find it particularly difficult at times when you're a doctor to deal with death and dying, especially when you first qualify. In the first postgraduate year, when you feel responsible for patients' lives for the first time, the earlier loss of a parent can sometimes be reawakened and felt keenly. Do make sure you have extra support at that time or whenever you experience any indications that your mood is going down. These feelings are rarely permanent and catching things early will often mean that depression is nipped in the bud.

> Michael was the first member of his family to go to university. His father had left the family home when he was a baby and, when he was in third year medicine and starting clinical work, his mother developed a brain tumour and died. Michael began drinking in earnest at her funeral and continued to drink heavily as it seemed to him an effective way of handling his grief. He now hated going onto wards, didn't want to talk to patients or socialise with other more enthusiastic medical students. He drank more and thought often about suicide. His frequent absences were noticed and the tutor began to talk to him about his mother. When he broke down, the tutor recognised his own limitations in handling this level of distress and referred him to a psychotherapist at the nearby hospital. Michael took a year out to tackle his alcohol use and to work through his grief and also the sense of guilt and failure that he felt, both that medicine was something he was doing for his mother, and because medicine had failed her. He resumed his studies but kept going to his psychotherapist throughout the undergraduate and first postgraduate year. He is now a senior consultant in psychiatry.

Heavy alcohol use (or using other drugs) by doctors is very frequently associated with depression, anxiety and, sadly, also with suicide. Although there's no doubt that many doctors say it seems to be a good way to tackle their stress early on, it gradually stops its effectiveness and life becomes more and more difficult to manage because of the alcohol rather than despite it. It may be that heavy alcohol use is a feature of depression, as in Michael's case, so that he needed to tackle both the depression and stop his drinking. However, sometimes it's an addiction to or dependence on alcohol or other drugs which leads to depression because of the way it gradually affects all aspects of your life. When you free yourself from this dependency, your mood lifts and life seems to start afresh. Chapter 9 deals with ways to do this.

Chronic tiredness from sleep loss is often overlooked as a precursor to depression. However, all the medical and military studies which look at the links between fatigue and performance consistently report that fatigue lowers your mood: if you're very tired because you've not had enough sleep you will feel sad and you won't perform as well as you should which then can lead to guilt and worry and bring your mood down even further. Add alcohol or other drugs to this equation and you're likely to find yourself on a slippery slope. With the reduction of working hours for doctors, it would be good to think that this cause of depression was a thing of the past. However, if the newly acquired time off is filled with looking after a new baby, or is used to party rather than to sleep, then you will quickly find yourself exhausted. It's not hours at work that matter – the policy-makers never read the evidence – it's hours of sleep, so make sure you get enough.

Doing less and less that gives you pleasure. When we're depressed we tend to lose energy and withdraw from things that would help. We don't go out so much, or talk to people, or visit the gym or dig the garden. Instead, we're more likely avoid a social life or to lie in bed and brood. Getting active again is a very important first step to changing things. There's no doubt that physical activity lifts mood and so going for a brisk walk or cleaning the house, visiting a gallery or swimming will all help: doing the things that give you pleasure does you good. When you're really low, you might need to get someone else to push you into this activity – a friend or a counsellor. Start small and build up to bigger things, and notice how your mood lifts when you do something. And put some extra pleasure back into your life – sit in the garden with a book, watch a movie that you've loved in the past, have a massage, learn to meditate: whatever works for you.

6.3 Keeping a diary

So that you know what works and what doesn't, start to keep a diary which provides a score for your mood before and after you do something. Writing things down helps to make everything clearer and provides a record for you to see what changes. Be the scientist that you are, and add a little more of what makes you feel good and a little less of what makes you feel bad. Once you've become more active and used to using a diary and assessing your mood in this way, start to write down the thoughts you've had in the same way. Take the thoughts 'I can never do anything right' and 'There's no point doing anything this book suggests as nothing will change'. Score how they make you feel: do they raise your mood or lower it? Well yes, it would be pretty surprising if they did anything but lowered it quite a lot. So you have to learn to challenge such negative thoughts and add positive ones, like listing all the things you've done right today, and telling yourself that you have nothing to lose by trying out some of these ideas about changing the way you think as the evidence has shown that this can help now and in the future. You could score your feelings again at this point. This thought-changing exercise needs a lot of practice but, as part of a CBT approach, has a good evidence base for reducing depression.

6.4 And when you're better

Most treatments for depression – whether psychotherapy, cognitive behaviour therapy or medication – have a reasonable success rate, and many episodes get better on their own or with self-help or by changing some aspect of our lives. Good! When this happens, however, it doesn't mean that you won't ever feel low again. All of us have bad days and even bad weeks, but this isn't a sign that means we've slipped back down into the pit that was depression. If you find yourself feeling low again, don't presume the worst; just realise that sometimes feeling sad is normal and that you now have plenty of useful strategies to start using at once: ways to stop the slippery slope while you're still on top.

6.5 Summary

- Remember that sadness and depression are a normal part of life, and everyone feels them at times. Realise that these are times to reflect and explore and to express some of the feelings that go with them.
- Get enough sleep.
- Get yourself moving. Plan in some physical activities each day even though it really seems an effort. Use a diary to find out which activities give you pleasures and which make you less happy, and plan into your day more of the former and less of the latter.
- Keep a thoughts diary. Write down negative thoughts and their effect on your mood, and then write alternatives to them and re-rate your mood.
- Don't treat stress or depression with alcohol or other drugs or with lots of food – not even in the short term. Dependency can strike fast when we are emotionally down.
- If you've lost someone, let yourself grieve. Don't get cross with yourself because you think you should be strong or because grief is taking too long. If you've lost someone in the past, see if there are links between that loss and what is happening to you now.
- Make sure you have some social support from a friend or a relative. If you feel these are lacking at the moment then get yourself a mentor or counsellor. At once!
- Recognise when you're angry and why, and find ways to dispel the anger. Bottled-up anger can be turned against yourself and become depression, and it's bad for your physical health too.
- Become your own best friend. Use some compassion on yourself and you'll find it easier to give it to others. Leave old criticisms and betrayals behind and learn to praise yourself and give yourself the rewards and treats that you deserve.

Bibliography

Center C, et al. Confronting depression and suicide in physicians: a consensus statement. *JAMA* 2003;**289**:3161–7.

Firth-Cozens J. Depression in doctors. In Katona, C & Robertson, MM (eds), *Depression and Physical Illness* (pp. 95–111). 1997, Wiley, Chichester.

Gilbert P. *Overcoming Depression: A Self-help Guide Using Cognitive Behavioral Techniques.* 2000, Robinson, London.

Isaksson Rø KE, Gude T, Tyssen R, Aasland OG. Counselling for burnout in Norwegian doctors: one year cohort study. *BMJ* 2008;**337**:a2004.

Williams M, *et al. The Mindful Way Through Depression.* 2007, Guildford Press, London.

Chapter 7 **Difficult people?**

The problem in dealing with difficult people in the workplace is that you can very rarely change them. Of course, if they are under you managerially, then you will usually have options to get them to toe the line as you want (perhaps) and we'll discuss that later. But usually it's more a matter that certain colleagues or patients wind you up the wrong way and you need to find ways to deal with that. The first option, and really the most important, is to look at yourself to see what part you play in the difficult transaction.

7.1 Could it be me?

When something goes wrong, everyone finds it difficult to look at the part they may have played in causing it to happen. From being toddlers we learn to argue furiously and with conviction why 'it wasn't me'. This happens even if we are deep down very self-critical; there's almost always a reaction to deny. But, if you want things to improve, it's worth considering the role you might be playing in difficult relationships.

Before you do anything else, find some time to sit down with a few blank sheets of paper. Draw a wide margin and, giving each item plenty of space, write the list of jobs you've had down the side, starting with the most recent. For each job write down someone – anyone – whom you found it hard to get on with. If you have a reason why this was difficult, write that down too. If you have time, do one for non-work relationships as well – people at university or clubs, those who you never liked, friends you made and finished with. Now write two lists of adjectives – all the things you most like in people, and all the things you dislike. Have a look at the four lists over a few days – if you have a partner or close friend, get them to look at it with you – and see if you can recognise any pattern in the type of people you dislike, who let you down,

---

or simply who get up your nose. Do you see them perhaps as over-authoritarian, untrustworthy, a bit cringing, too full of themselves, corner-cutters, bullies, arrogant, needy or anything else you come up with. Are they usually women, or usually men? What you're looking for is a pattern – anything that pops up a few times, maybe anything that fits what you've written in the list of pet hates, or maybe you find you're adding to it as you work.

There are all sorts of reasons why we find particular types of people more difficult to get on with – reasons beyond the obvious one that some people simply rub *everyone* up the wrong way. We'll deal here with three that can cause definite problems.

1 **Mood.** It's always worth thinking first about your mood in general. Are you stressed or depressed? Ask a friend or someone close if you're not sure. Because if your mood is low you will probably be irritable or at least see things in a much more negative light. So you might see criticism where it's simply reasonable feedback, while people who are genuinely irritating become much more difficult to tolerate. As we've described earlier, self-critical people can often be very sensitive to what they see as criticism and may come across as even belligerent in defending themselves, and self-criticism is highly related to depression. If low mood might be a factor, use the strategies in Chapters 5 and 6 to help yourself, or get help from your doctor.
2 **Type differences.** If you remind yourself of the different dimensions of the MBTI described in Chapter 2, you will see that dealing with individuals who are not your type on any dimension might at times prove irritating:
   - On the **Extraversion–Introversion (E–I)** dimension, people who are Es can find it difficult to know what Is think about anything. Whereas some Es let you know straight away what they think, and argue through their decisions verbally, Is like to think about things first and so it sometimes feels as if they are being almost belligerently silent. Of course, Is may find Es noisy, verbose and inappropriately open about everything: they don't always want to hear a life history in the first five minutes. Es sometimes think that Is are neurotic, but they're not; they're just different in the ways they process things and live their lives. Is need to tell Es that they would like to think about that – actually say the words so they can understand. Es need to realise that they are dealing with differences and curb their noise and their anecdotes as much as possible. We can all act like the other end of the dimension, so try it now and then see the effects.
   - On the **Sensing–Intuitive (S–N)** dimension, Ss often find Ns woolly and even frighteningly chaotic in the way they deal with things: ignoring the facts before them and making leaps beyond the evidence. Ns can be irritated by the way an S seems to hold them back, goes on about the past

or the data, fails to think enough about the future. But once difference is appreciated, Ss and Ns can work together marvellously because they realise what they do will be much better as a combination.

- The **Thinking–Feeling (T–F)** dimension causes the most problems as we described earlier. While Ts realise that they don't have to like everyone they work with, Fs find it upsetting if everyone fails to be in harmony. They dislike what they see as conflict and are more easily hurt than Ts. Ts don't see an interaction as conflict until much later, and enjoy a strong debate. They are blunt sometimes to the point of tactlessness. They will often describe Fs as being too needy, or as giving poor feedback, not realising that Fs are being over-careful not to hurt anyone's feelings. Ts have a very strong sense of justice and so will sometimes carry on making a point or finding 'the truth' long after it might be better to let it go. Again, it's about appreciating the two types – that logic and justice matter, but so do people and harmony.
- The **Judgment–Process (J–P)** dimension can cause irritations too, but not real conflict. Js like to make their decisions fast, whereas Ps dilly-dally if they are allowed. Js seem much more organised too and prepare for meetings way in advance, while Ps might want the meeting itself to be a preparation for something else. Nevertheless, we need Ps to make sure we don't make decisions too fast, and Js to make sure we make one at all.

Matthew was an ISFP and a registrar in neurology. He was asked to get coaching for unprofessional behaviour – shouting down a senior surgeon, and arguing with a colleague in front of a patient. In each case, he said, what he did was later shown to be for the patient's benefit. He had checked with the nurses and they had said he was right. It was clear that he cared passionately about the welfare of patients and felt that his colleagues cut corners. It turned out that he spent more time with the nursing staff than with the doctors. The coach reminded him that, unlike him, most doctors were Ts and most nurses were Fs so that, when talking to doctors he needed to stay rational, provide the evidence rather than anything emotive. He should speak up sooner rather than stay silent till he was really angry. And, rather than use nurses as a retreat, he needed to learn how to handle his peers, listen to the way they talked and made decisions, and develop his skills of rational persuasion.

3 **Family matters.** There have been a number of longitudinal studies of doctors which have shown that your early family relationships have an effect on various aspects of your wellbeing, mood and relationships. For example, one of the principal stressors for general practitioners concerns their relationships with their partners, usually to do with a perceived inequality in terms of time or

desirable roles. But in addition, one of the main predictors of their stress is if they reported (many years earlier) an envious relationship with their siblings.[1] It seems that the old inequalities seen as a child were being relived in the new situation of the practice and causing problems for some of the partners.

It is always worth thinking about your parents and siblings if you find that there is a pattern of dislike for a particular type of person – or even anyone in authority or someone who consistently makes you feel inadequate or guilty. Think about whether they remind you of a parent, how you used to feel as a child in that relationship and whether you feel similar today. These child–adult reverberations are the essence of psychotherapy and some of you might decide that that would be a useful route. However, many people can move past these old ties and memories simply by getting insight into how they have developed.

Matthew, described above, also talked about his bullying aggressive father and how he'd tried and failed to stand up against him when he reduced his mother to tears, as he often did. Part of the changes that Matthew was able to make in terms of his relationships at work was to do with the realisation that he often saw authority figures as aggressive and uncaring, and that some of that probably belonged in the past.

7.2 Dealing with difficult people

One factor within emotional intelligence is that you have developed a reasonable understanding of yourself. The more you can appreciate about yourself – your mood, your personality and any baggage you might bring from earlier times – the better you will get on with people. However, the other aspect of emotional intelligence is that you are able to understand other people so that you have reasonable explanations for why they are behaving the way they are and can vary your own reactions and behaviour appropriately. Altering your perceptions of the problem can help a lot. Here are some strategies for developing this understanding and for dealing with people who seem (and you've checked this out with reliable others) really difficult to deal with.

Other-consciousness. We all know about self-consciousness – feeling scrutinised, embarrassed, possibly found lacking – especially in situations of evaluation like interviews or feedback sessions. Other-consciousness is useful in these situations but also when someone seems aggressive or unreasonable. It involves you looking squarely at the person and starting to think

[1]Firth-Cozens J. Individual and organizational predictors of depression in general practitioners. Br J Gen Pract 1998;**48**:1647–51.

about him, her or them. Do they look well or ill or tired; why might they be irritable (problems at home? frustrations at work? depressed?); who are they trying to impress or what are the relationships between him/her and the others? And so on. Turn yourself into an observant psychologist for a moment; this takes your scrutiny off yourself and helps you to relate to the difficult other person in a warmer, more understanding way that changes the situation for the better.

Empathy and action. In the early 1980s one of the housing departments in the East London boroughs had a real violence problem and no houses. Each day desperate people came up against officers who couldn't help but appeared confrontational in reporting this. A consultant taught them to empathise: 'It must be dreadful for you and your family in that bedsit. I really wish I could help.' Violence vanished over night. If you can empathise with the person, after you've tried to understand them, so much the better, especially if it's followed by potential offers to improve things. Statements like, 'Running this department must be a nightmare sometimes', or 'You must sometimes feel a bit overwhelmed with all this responsibility', 'Tough day?' or 'I think I'm being a bit slow to get on top of this. Hope I'm not driving you mad!' You can follow any of these types of statements by questions such as 'Is there anything I can do to help?', or 'Can you suggest some steps for me to take?'

Managing disagreement. Medicine is full of uncertainty and there are many areas where you might have to argue your point. If you feel that a discussion is turning into a disagreement there are a series of steps to take that often help, based on what we've said above. First, manage yourself: check your body for tension and cool it with some deep breaths and calm thoughts. If you practise relaxation or meditation, this is easy. Summarise the discussion so far and check that they see it in that way too; then ask what would change their view. Take an 'other-consciousness' stance when they tell you: are there any emotions attached to what they say? Is this something more than a technical argument? Let them know you understand and recognise their concerns and then tell them what, if anything, you will do to help meet them. If you have things you'd like them to do to test out your side of the argument, this is the time to state them clearly. Summarise what both of you have agreed to do and, depending on the outcome, what the next steps might be.

If the disagreement has gone too far already and you feel like shouting or crying, then it's always better to take some time out and cool down. Tell them you would like to think about this more and suggest you meet later to continue the discussion. Then take a walk round the block (whatever your 'block' happens to be, but preferably outside) or go somewhere quiet and do a few relaxation exercises. There is never any point trying to win a disagreement when you're caught emotionally.

7.3 The bully and the bullied

Bullying is said to be rife in health care as it is in many other types of organisation.

There are two types of people accused of bullying in the workplace: those who intend to hurt and who pick their victims in order to get pleasure or excitement from using their power – and they should be complained about at once – and those where the accusation of bullying is linked to a disagreement over what represents normal social behaviour. The accuser feels bullied by behaviour the accused sees as reasonable. In turn, the accused may feel bullied by the strong reaction of the accuser to what they themselves see as a normal interaction; they often suffer as hard a blow to their self-esteem as the one who has claimed the status of victim. Medicine occurs within an arena of uncertainty where right and wrong sometimes have a variety of perspectives, and so the chance for disagreements such as these is likely to be high, particularly when the outcome of being wrong can cause such damage.

In reality, one person's bullying is another's tough management. Senior doctors and trainers must be able to direct others to perform their duties in particular ways, and to stop them doing things badly, but equally they can be questioned about their orders and be able to discuss their reasons. If you feel bullied it's worth doing the exercise at the beginning to see whether there has been any pattern of this throughout your working life or before it. Are you playing any part in it and, if so, can you change things, perhaps by using some of the techniques described above? This is a difficult area and one where assertive training from a coach or an exploration of the pattern with a psychotherapist can both be particularly useful.

In fact, there are many reasons why these interactions can lead to accusations and counter-accusations. First, consider (whichever side you are on) that you might be involved in a T–F interaction – that the apparently critical and tactless T doesn't realise that the other is different, an F who expected a harmonious and careful relationship to exist. Second, there is relatively little training in management or leadership skills provided for doctors and they may not always express their authority tactfully. Newly appointed consultants are expected to take over complex multi-disciplinary teams, revolutionise service delivery, and become excellent trainers almost overnight and this is unreasonable and probably impossible to do well. As a new consultant or partner you need management development and support so you don't feel bound to model yourself on the outmoded styles of your own trainers, or be unduly harsh in your anxiety to exert control.

Most doctors accused of bullying feel astounded that their behaviour is being interpreted in this way. This can evoke a defensive – even combative – response which is not helpful. If a colleague informally expresses the feeling that you are bullying or harassing them, it is wise to respond positively and take the information seriously. Many cases can be resolved if the aggrieved parties feel that their concerns have been listened to and that change has resulted. It might be difficult, but be grateful that you have been given the opportunity to sort things out and seriously consider how you might modify your behaviour. Coaching and any opportunity you have to get 360° feedback from your colleagues will help you do this.

7.4 Treating other doctors

Finally, as we said in Chapter 1, it's often very difficult to treat other doctors or their relatives. Doctors don't make good patients and it's wise to recognise that they might not be giving you all the facts about themselves simply because they don't want the diagnosis they suspect. It is stressful to treat someone you know well, especially when that person is a colleague, so at least discuss the problem with a mentor or see if your colleague will agree to getting help elsewhere. It is important not to go along with their reluctance to be ill and to get them to agree that they will not treat themselves as well as being treated by you.

I worked in a large GP practice where two of the GPs consulted each other over medical matters. At one point both became unwell and issued sickness absence notes for each other. This caused quite a few problems for the practice.

The same applies where the doctor concerned works in the same GP practice, especially if he or she is a medical partner. It's important to make sure that all GPs have their own general practitioner in a neighbouring practice, someone who can act impartially and wisely in giving proper clinical advice to the doctor–patient concerned.

7.5 Conclusion

Many of us feel we should like everyone we work with in order for there to be harmony. That might be nice but liking everyone is impossible. Moreover, as Blake told us, 'without contraries is no progression': we need the rubbing up against others occasionally in order to do something new that's hopefully better. Conflict that is worked with is productive. We sometimes even make leaps forward in understanding ourselves by dealing well with people that we would rather avoid. So work at it: it can be fruitful.

Bibliography

Berger AS. Arrogance among physicians. Acad Med 2002;**77**:145–7.

De Bono E. *Conflicts: A Better Way to Resolve Them*. 1986, Penguin, London.

Ingstad B, Christie VM. Encounters with illness: the perspective of the sick doctor. *Anthropol Med* 2001;**8**:201–10.

Keirsey D, Bates M. *Please Understand Me: Character & Temperament Types*. 1984, Prometheus Nemesis Book Company, Del Mar.

Margerison, CJ. *If Only I Had Said…* 1990, Mercury, London.

Paice E, Aitken M, Houghton A, Firth-Cozens J. Bullying among doctors in training: Paice E, Firth-Cozens J., Who's a bully then? *BMJ*, 2003;**326**:S127, cross sectional questionnaire survey. *BMJ* 2004;**329:**658–659.

Paice E, Firth-Cozens J. Who's bully then? *BMJ*, 2003; 326:S127.

Rodenburg P. *Presence: How to Use Positive Energy for Success in Every Situation*. 2007, Michael Joseph, London.

Chapter 8 **Feeling angry**

Contrary to some popular myths, anger is not good for you – poor for relationships, deadly for your heart and draining away so much of the energy you might use in other more enjoyable ways. Whether your anger appears in frequent short bursts of rage or is part of long-standing resentments, yearnings for revenge, or outrage at perceived injustices, the emotion will do you little good and may cause you harm in your careers, your health and your personal life. If anger is never or rarely something you experience, you might want to skip this chapter, unless perhaps you know someone at work or home who might benefit from your knowledge.

History is a catalogue of angry men, often urged on by angry women, taking out their rage on other religions, other races, other nations. Outbursts of rage are one indicator of low emotional intelligence: those with high emotional intelligence are able to use their emotions well rather than destructively. The work of Paice and Orton at the London Deanery shows that what they term 'ward rage' is an important indicator of a doctor in difficulty. Doctors who are socially intelligent – able to manage their emotions and interactions in order to bring about the best solution – are also likely to have a good effect on their patients and to keep them and their carers calm instead of building up tension and accusations.

But anger is a normal emotion and bottling it up has been linked to arthritis and depression. On the other hand, feeling constantly hostile and letting it go at random contributes most to the behaviours called Type A that are seen as contributing to heart disease. There is no doubt that it is very important to recognise as early as possible that you feel angry, appreciate the deeper causes of it rather than just the superficial and immediate, and do something constructive to deal with it. So, if you look back to the case of

Matthew (Chapter 7), he was able to realise that his rage against the consultant and others in authority happened so regularly that it was likely to represent something bigger and more fundamental in the attitudes he held about authority figures and his need to protect more vulnerable others from what he saw as their cruelty. Seeing the links between his workplace relationships and those of his parents set him on the road to change. This is not to say that the care he saw the other doctors give was necessarily good – sometimes it may not have been even close – but in reacting with anger he became seen as someone who was not best able to say how things were, so could have no effect on future quality: he failed to help the patient and he ended up disciplined with the real potential of having to leave medicine. If you see injustices and poor care that you want to end, then handling it carefully without anger will be a much better route.

8.1 Analysing your anger

The sooner you realise that you feel angry, or even just irritable, the better it is. As cavemen, angry feelings were undoubtedly so vital in dealing immediately with the enemy that attacked you that they are still one of the fastest emotions to get out of control. But you're rarely going to be faced with anything quite so dangerous nowadays, and so you need to be prepared to catch the emotion as early as you can. You'll learn to do that sooner if you practise any means of recognising what is happening in your body and mind; for example, through relaxation or through mindfulness meditation. Practise being open about your feelings to members of your family, and learn to accept their honesty about what they feel too. This will stop anger building up. Doing this at work needs more careful handling and is better done as part of a structured mutual feedback session or regular team meeting – not in the corridor!

When you appreciate those signs and symptoms of anger, try to think about what has caused this at work today. Here's some of the simpler suggestions:

- You slept badly last night.
- You're hungry.
- You're concerned about what your adolescent son is getting up to (it isn't his homework!).
- The bills that arrived this morning made you worried you had bitten off too much.
- You suspect the dry rot is back.
- You had a row with your partner.

These are a few of the hundreds of common reasons why you might feel stressed and grumpy at work, despite the fact that the culprits are elsewhere, so deal with them at source rather than in the workplace. Realising where they belong relieves you of what you felt towards colleagues or patients.

Then there are more complicated reasons that take more time and greater patience, and sometimes outside help, to appreciate:

- The way your senior doctor or manager spoke to you made you feel like a child. But then, for example, you think about the way your father spoke to you; perhaps how he used his strength to belittle you and you realise that this has become a common reaction to someone's feedback or apparent criticism.
- There is a particular partner in the practice who infuriates you. She always seems to see fewer patients than anyone else and gets out of many of the things you see as chores. But then you think about when you had this feeling before and realise that these infuriated, envious thoughts were a common part of your reactions to a sibling you saw as favoured. Perhaps your partner is as lazy and selfish as you see her, but the real anger belongs long ago and dealing just with her won't abolish it.
- You have exploded at a fairly small request or error by a colleague. You feel guilty at your reaction and that makes you feel even more angry. When you think about it more carefully you realise that it's just the last straw in a long line of people who ask you constantly to do things for them or fix things when they do them wrong – maybe a partner, a mother, your children, your girlfriend or boyfriend, the neighbours… Not to mention the patients. Sometimes we give and give in the hope that we might get something back from others and we can from time to time explode when nothing seems to come our way. But the explosion belongs in the past – perhaps to when we tried and tried to make a parent happy – rather than the poor person who asked you for something simple today.

You can sometimes recognise these early causes of anger or distress by the following exercise.

Sit somewhere quiet, shut your eyes and relax as much as you can. Now think of yourself as a child walking up to the door of your home, opening it and looking round. Take your time. Now see your mother (if she was there) and notice what she's doing as you come in. How does she greet you? And now your father – how does he greet you? Take some time to think about this. Now imagine that you have done something good at school. What do they each say to you? Who shows you appreciation and how do they do it? What if you've not done so well at something? Again, what does each of them say to you? What do they do? Take your time, and when you've finished write down anything you've discovered and how it might affect the way you respond to others at work.

Recognising possible root causes of your anger – or at least realising that sometimes it might not be to do with the current situation but to something that happened earlier – is one way to reappraise it and let it go: to decide that, although this person or situation might be very irritating, the real anger or upset that you feel perhaps belongs to a time when you never seemed to do anything right for a parent.

Another means of reappraisal is by practising 'other-consciousness' (see Chapter 7) and empathy with the person making you angry: focussing on them and realising what they might be experiencing at the moment. Perhaps you can talk to them to see if anything is going wrong in their lives. This exterior focus (rather than on you, the victim) can often help a lot in putting out the flames. Thinking about the reasonable compact you have made with your employers (see Chapter 10) again might be useful in some circumstances; for example, where the burdens on you seem to be unfair.

8.2 Anger and depression

Many of the examples above may well happen when you're depressed. Irritability is an accepted symptom of depression, anxiety and PTSD, so take these possibilities into your analysis. When you are depressed you will often feel angry – even destructively so – towards yourself, and sometimes this anger gets directed towards other people instead or as well.

> When Margaret's husband left her with two small children and took a consultant's job elsewhere, her rage knew no bounds. She ranted away about him to friends, but also exploded at work with colleagues who were trying to support her. At home she was far from the sort of mother she wanted to be for her children. She knew she was being horrible at times and felt terribly guilty about it. She also felt that perhaps she was to blame for the separation – that she hadn't been caring enough in the marriage, that she wasn't slim enough, sexy enough, etc. When she talked about her anger she said that she needed it just to keep the awful sadness away – that a black hole of despair was lurking there underneath: anger made her feel in control while sadness might wash her away. It was only when she got in touch with her sadness and let herself cry properly that her feelings of rage began to diminish.

So think about sadness and loss when you find yourself feeling angry a lot and scattering it around in a random sort of way. Sadness needs dealing with if you are to escape from the grips of a simmering rage. Even if you feel angry with someone in the present, still think about the past. Here is a very useful exercise for exorcising those early demons:

> *Write a letter or speak into a tape-recorder saying what you wished you'd said to some significant other – maybe a partner, maybe a parent who's now died or too old to hear it. Notice how you feel as you speak or write. Alternatively, stand and focus on an empty chair and imagine the person in that. Notice how you feel as you look down on that person, and what your body's doing as you speak. Whether you're writing or speaking, try to use powerful phrases beginning with 'I'; for example, 'I resent you for…', 'I hate you for…', rather than weak victim phrases like: 'You did that to me'. If it's difficult to say or write the words, notice what it feel like physically to hold it in. If you're using an empty chair and feel like pounding it with a rolled up newspaper, do so, but make sure you don't hurt yourself: chances are you're pretty good at that! When you feel finished for the day, say goodbye. That's important. You can always bring them back again whenever you want. If this seems too difficult to do alone, someone who is trained in gestalt psychotherapy may help you through it.*

8.3 Cooling down

If you're too over-heated to even begin to analyse or re-think what is happening, then you need to find physical ways to cool down fast. Ventilating your anger doesn't work at all; in fact research has shown that it raises your emotional state rather than cooling you down. And it gets you into trouble and takes away support from those around you. Even taking what seems like justified revenge against the right person doesn't help: you hear people telling you about their wonderful methods of getting their own back, but you can see at once that it hasn't taken away their anger one little bit. If it did, they wouldn't need to repeat it over and over.

If you can, leave the situation and take yourself outside. Walk or run round the 'block' – real or metaphorical – if that's possible; go down to the chapel if you're in a hospital; or put yourself in a room on your own and do a few energetic exercises or a brief relaxation. Some form of exercise takes the edge off anger, but relaxation will do the same. If you are skilled at it (and you will be if you practise it often) you will find you don't need to leave the room but can simply check your body over, find out where it's tense and trying to explode and relax it bit by bit. If you use a mantra of some sort when you practise, then say that to yourself now. This is a skill that will help you through all sorts of difficult situations all through your life, so don't ignore it just because it's simple.

Most of the remedies and exercises in the chapters on stress and depression and dealing with difficult people will also work well for dealing with anger (Chapters 5–7). Greater self-awareness will help you to understand why you flare up and how to work out strategies to avoid confrontations with colleagues and complaints from patients. However much you think your team is hopeless or your patient condescending, informing them of your views will not help them or you. There are usually much more successful ways to bring about change or to accept what can't, at the moment, be altered.

Bibliography

Cozens J. *OK2 Talk Feelings*. 1991, BBC Books, London.

Harbin T. *Beyond Anger: A Guide for Men*. 2000, Marlowe & Co., London.

Semmelroth C, Smith D. *The Anger Habit: Proven Principles to Calm the Stormy Mind*. 2004, Sourcebooks Inc., Naperville.

Chapter 9 **A little too much**

Alcohol is a particular problem for doctors – one that has been recognised for decades. This is true whether we measure it by their psychiatric admissions or by their cirrhotic deaths. Professionals as a whole drink more than others, partly due to earning more, but most studies show that doctors consume the most. It is largely a hidden problem with doctors taking many years to admit to addiction and their colleagues being slow to confront it so that, by the time it becomes public, the effects on the doctor's career or health or patients can be devastating.

During medical school alcohol intake stays around the same despite entering the clinical years. In fact, it even rises for women, whereas for other women students it falls over the years. In addition, women doctors are more likely than male colleagues to use alcohol to cope with their stress and depression, and its links to suicide are considerable. As you no doubt know, alcohol affects your physical health as well with most organs of your body, including your brain, reeling from the effects of too much too often, while your relationships, including your sex life, suffer sometimes permanent damage.

Doctors in different specialties vary considerably, however, in having problems. Surgeons have the lowest rates of substance abuse, but also are the least stressed and depressed (see Chapter 4). Most studies show psychiatrists to have the highest levels, but those in emergency medicine and family or general practitioners are also seen as having high rates. In terms of illegal drug use, opioids are most commonly used by those in emergency medicine and by anaesthetists who also show high fentanyl use. Benzodiazepines seem to be the drug of choice for psychiatrists. Consultants show more alcohol dependency than non-consultants who are more likely to use other drugs, especially cocaine, cannabis and benzodiazepines: perhaps a generation issue. In one UK study around a third of addicted doctors were abusing both alcohol and drugs.

In terms of drugs other than alcohol, doctors in 1988 were found to be between 30 and 100 times more likely to become addicted to narcotics than the general population, though today, with heroin and cocaine use becoming so common, it's likely that the general population has at least caught up. Drug dependency in doctors has been reported as high in the United Kingdom, the United States, Europe and Australia; for example, one Australian State programme for impaired doctors reported 45% of referrals were for drug misuse while only 7% were for alcohol. Illegal drug use in doctors may, it seems, be growing as younger doctors choose this rather than alcohol. Since doctors who are addicted usually misappropriate their drugs from the workplace, this creates a particular problem for health services.

Most students and young people drink more than they should for their health and their work, but most young professionals other than doctors have enough time and a regular working life to enable them to begin to develop ways to cope with their stress other than by using alcohol or other drugs. Now that working hours have been shortened in many countries, you might think that the problem would be less as young doctors use their spare time for sport or families or start to develop new hobbies. However, at the same time as hours reduced, society has taken on a new level of alcohol and drug dependence and this is unlikely to have missed the leisure time of the medical profession. As we've seen earlier, stress and depression are common in medicine and using any drugs, including alcohol, as a way to cope is dangerous to you and to your patients as these quotes from a young anaesthetist and an emergency medicine consultant show:

> *I am so tired so often that I just want to collapse in a chair and have a few drinks. This causes shaky hands the next day, so epidurals etc are more difficult.*

> *The day often gets to me: something goes wrong and I keep thinking did I do all I could, and I find the easiest way to block it out is by having a few drinks.*

9.1 Is it a problem for you?

There are many simple ways of judging whether or not you are a problem drinker or an alcoholic. The simplest way is called 'The Four Ls': if your Liver, or your Lover (partners, family or friends), or your Labour, or your dealings with the Law (losing your Licence, getting into fights) has been affected by drugs or alcohol, then you have a problem. We could add 'your Lucre', as the financial costs of addiction are obviously huge. Most of these indicators will be just as affected in addiction to other drugs. There is another short test with a much stronger scientific basis at the end of the chapter.

It's not difficult to substitute some of these questions for drug use. If anyone ever suggests to you that you might have a problem, whether with drugs or alcohol, take it very seriously: it requires a lot of courage for a friend or colleague to say this, and chances are you have some level of problem if they do. And if they do, don't then go around all your hard-drinking friends or fellow drug users to ask for confirmation that really you are fine: they will say 'Yes, you're perfectly normal', but it's a completely unreliable test of dependency. And don't think that, just because you can stop completely for even weeks at a time that you are not an alcoholic if, when you do start drinking you drink on and on: 'I'm not dependent; I'm only a binge drinker' is nonsense. But people say it. The problem with illegal drugs is, by the time you come to test out whether you can stop or not, chances are you will already be addicted. In the United Kingdom, the Sick Doctors Trust is staffed by volunteer doctors, some of whom have had alcohol or drug problems but who have been sober or clean for decades. They should be able to help you decide.

If after all this you still are unsure whether or not you have a problem, take yourself to an Alcoholics Anonymous (AA) meeting or a Narcotics Anonymous (NA) meeting. The stories the members tell will help you make up your mind and the members themselves are usually very capable of judging if you ask them. Your general practitioner is unlikely to be as good at this: doctors are very wary of diagnosing dependency in any of their patients, perhaps worrying about their own levels of consumption. In the United States, where there is routine or random screening for alcohol and drug misuse in organisations, recognition isn't a problem and treatment for those who need it is widely available.

9.2 Tackling addiction

Like most psychological problems, this one is better recognised and tackled early. However, most people's experience shows that the addiction is well established by the time they acknowledge that stopping has become difficult. Addiction is a love affair: it takes you over so that you get to think and do little that isn't linked to it. Because of this, when you stop you are bereft initially: your life is empty and socialising is difficult. Recovery has to provide the type of support which will take this into account. In terms of alcohol, Britain, as opposed to the United States, still favours 'controlled drinking' as the principal intervention. In this you use various psychological strategies, such as cognitive behavioural techniques, to learn how to stop after one or two drinks. Most people will try some form of controlled drinking for a while before admitting that, for a substantial proportion of them, total freedom from alcohol is the only way.

In terms of other drugs, you are unlikely to find that mental health workers will suggest controlled use, that an occasional dose of heroin or benzodiazepines is safe, though methadone is commonly prescribed. For doctors abstinence is the only safe route, and the most successful way to achieve this freedom is by joining AA or NA; in fact one of the first two members of AA was a doctor! Most rehabilitation clinics use the 12-step approach of AA and, for self-help, AA meetings attended only by doctors also exist in most countries. Doctors generally do unusually well in treatment or in AA or NA; for example, the Sick Doctors' Trust found relapse rates of only 4% at a five-year follow-up. In a US study around a quarter had at least one relapse, particularly if there was a family history of substance abuse, or doctors were also using a major opioid. Doctors rarely make good patients and this is certainly an area where all their antagonisms towards being helped rather than being a helper can come to the fore, particularly in the case of psychiatrists. So it helps to recognise this in yourself early on if you are going to do well.

Addiction services specially designed for doctors are available in the United States, the United Kingdom, Spain and Australia: some are private and some provided by the local health service. Doctors who voluntarily contract with a practitioner/physician health programme (PHP) will usually be allowed to remain anonymous and this encourages earlier interventions. But in some cases the problem has gone too far and disciplinary boards such as the General Medical Council become involved. This is by no means the end of the line for a doctor as it might be just the 'rock bottom' needed to prompt rehabilitation and eventually a return to work, fully back on track. There is no one route to freedom from addiction, but whatever way you choose to do it, remember that the first AA step is the most important and probably the hardest: 'We admitted we were powerless over alcohol – that our lives had become unmanageable.' Once you're on that step you're on the road to recovery.

Sylvia was a high-flyer through medical school and landed a good teaching hospital post when she graduated. She had always been a formidable drinker, 'easily able to keep up with the boys'. In her first post-graduate year she suffered a panic attack and began to take benzodiazepines as well as continuing to drink heavily. This seemed to control the inevitable stress she was experiencing with very long hours and a competitive, harsh medical environment. When she came to work one morning clearly still inebriated the registrar sent her home but didn't report her because 'we've all been there at some point'. He did her no favours. The next year she added cocaine to her list and then found herself in a psychiatric hospital with what looked like mania. She was eventually suspended by the GMC who appointed a medical supervisor for her. This doctor helped her to organise her rehabilitation and to start going to NA and AA meetings regularly, and also to a group for addicted doctors. This support, and the realisation that this was a last chance to get her career back on track, has kept her clean and sober since then.

The Alcohol Use Disorders Identification Test: Interview Version.	
1. How often do you have a drink containing alcohol?	0 points - Never 1 point - Monthly or less 2 points - 2 to 4 times a MONTH 3 points - 2 to 3 times a WEEK 4 points - 4 or more times a week
Questioner may skip to Questions 9 and 10 if reply to Question 1 is never, or if both answers to Q 2 and 3 are 0.	
2. How many drinks containing alcohol do you have on a typical day when you are drinking?	0 points - 1 or 2 drinks 1 point - 3 or 4 drinks 2 points - 5 or 6 drinks 3 points - 7 or 8 or 9 drinks 4 points - 10 or more drinks
3. How often do you have six or more drinks on one occasion?	0 points - Never 1 point - Less than monthly 2 points - Monthly 3 points - Weekly 4 points - Daily or almost daily
AUDIT-C Score ☐ /12 (complete full questionnaire if score is 3 or more)	
4. How often during the last year have you found that you were not able to stop drinking once you had started?	0 points - Never 1 point - Less than monthly 2 points - Monthly 3 points - Weekly 4 points - Daily or almost daily

Figure 9.1 The AUDIT TOOL. AUDIT was tested on a sample of 913 drinking patients, and has 92% sensitivity and specificity of 94% using the ≥8/40 threshold. The AUDIT-C is a shortened version of the above using the first three questions only. Using a cut-off ≥4 the AUDIT-C has a sensitivity of 86% of patients with heavy drinking and/or active alcohol abuse or dependence with a specificity of 72%. Using a cut-off of ≥3, AUDIT-C identifies 90% of patients with active alcohol abuse or dependence and 98% of patients with heavy drinking (specificity was only 60%, false-positive rate 40%). It is recommended a score of ≥3 or more points on the AUDIT-C, or a report of drinking 6 or more drinks on one occasion ever in the last year, should lead to a more detailed assessment of drinking and related problems.

5. How often during the last year have you failed to do what was normally expected from you because of drinking?	0 points - Never 1 point - Less than monthly 2 points - Monthly 3 points - Weekly 4 points - Daily or almost daily
6. How often during the last year have you needed a first drink in the morning to get yourself going after a heavy drinking session?	0 points - Never 1 point - Less than monthly 2 points - Monthly 3 points - Weekly 4 points - Daily or almost daily
7. How often during the last year have you had a feeling of guilt or remorse after drinking?	0 points - Never 1 point - Less than monthly 2 points - Monthly 3 points - Weekly 4 points - Daily or almost daily
8. How often during the last year have you been unable to remember what happened the night before because you had been drinking?	0 points - Never 1 point - Less than monthly 2 points - Monthly 3 points - Weekly 4 points - Daily or almost daily
9. Have you or someone else been injured as a result of your drinking?	0 points - No, never 2 points - Yes, but not in the last year 4 points - Yes, during the last year
10. Has a relative or friend or a doctor or another health worker been concerned about your drinking or suggested you cut down?	0 points - No, never 2 points - Yes, but not in the last year 4 points - Yes, during the last year
The Alcohol Use Disorders Identification Test (AUDIT) Score = /40	

Scores of 8 or more are considered an indicator of hazardous and harmful alcohol use. Reset

Figure 9.1 *(Continued)*

Bibliography

The AUDIT TOOL: (http://www.patient.co.uk/showdoc/40026159).

Ghodse H, et al. *Doctors and Their Health.* 2000, Centre for Addiction Studies, St George's Medical School, London.

Ghodse H, *Addiction at Work: Tackling Drug Use and Misuse in the Workplace.* 2005, Gower Publishing Ltd, Eldershot England, Burlington, USA.

Hughes PH, Brandenburg N, Baldwin DC, et al. Prevalence of substance use among US physicians. *JAMA* 1992;**267**:2333–9.

Khantzian EJ, Mack JE. How AA works and why it's important for clinicians to understand. *J Subst Abuse Treat* 1994;**11**:77–92.

Mayall R. Helping addicted doctors. *BMJ Career Focus* 2006;**333**:125.

McLellan AT, Skipper GS, Campbell M, DuPont RL. Five year outcomes in a cohort study of physicians treated for substance use disorders in the United States, *BMJ* 2008;**337**:a2038.

Chapter 10 **Demands, demands, demands!**

Medicine is a demanding occupation. The training is long and sometimes arduous and you are faced with evaluations that last right through your career – formal ones from the profession and informal ones from patients. Patients have always wanted a physician to take them seriously and deal with their problems and they don't always understand that you can't do magic. They often come to you when they are stressed and worried and so not at their most reasonable. Nowadays governments add considerably to these pressures by applying their own targets and directives which don't always seem to be in line with the type of care you think is best.

So anyone setting off on a career in medicine needs to be warned that the future will pose all sorts of demands and complexities. These will inevitably test your stamina, concentration and goodwill towards your fellow human beings. There will be times when the demands seem overwhelming and you wonder if you shouldn't just give up on medicine. This chapter offers ways of understanding and managing demands and then illustrates these throughout your career.

10.1 Strategies to make life easier

1 **A healthy lifestyle.** There is no doubt at all that you will work better, and feel better about your work, if you stay healthy. This means paying attention to diet, exercise, alcohol consumption and sleep. A lack of sleep lowers mood, memory and concentration which means every task will take longer, be done less well and will leave you feeling less satisfied. All those stressors and life events listed in Chapter 2 – the death of a young patient, apparently poor feedback from your boss, an argument with your partner – will

affect you more if you are exhausted. And if you get irritable when you're tired (and most people do), then you might drive away the very support you need. Burning a candle at both ends doesn't make a lovely light, whatever the poets might suggest.

2 **Managing your thoughts.** It might seem strange that demands can be reduced by the way you think, but they can. What is asked of you remains the same, of course, but your feelings about it change. Sometimes it happens without effort – you wake up and all day you see everything as easy – but when it doesn't, there are all sorts of cognitive strategies to cope with demands. For example:
   - *Relaxation.* If you learn a relaxation skill and practise it well you will find that you can use it whenever you feel under pressure. That's good for you physically, but it can also have the effect of changing how you think about things. For example, one young doctor told us:

   'I was way behind this morning and the nurses seemed to be getting impatient. I started to put a line in a cancer patient whose veins were really flat and difficult. He flinched and I thought 'This is mad' and I stopped. I began to talk to him as a person instead of a chore, at the same time thinking about where my body was tense and just letting it go. When I felt better the line went in perfectly and I found myself thinking about what was still to do in a much more organised and positive way. I've always been pleased I learnt relaxation – it comes in useful over and over.'

   - *Positive comparisons.* When you're feeling overwhelmed it helps to focus on what really matters. Watching the news and thinking how well off you are compared to almost anyone in the world in the latest disaster zone can put the demands into perspective.
   - *This is it.* The Buddhists recommend we realise that this is life, rather than fighting it all the time or looking for more. In terms of demands, 'this is it' can sometimes stop you constantly looking for completion, for the end of an overwhelming number of chores which in fact will never end because that's the job. This is particularly frustrating for Js (see the MBTI section of Chapter 2) who like to finish things. For them, and for most of us, it's better to think of each task separately, enjoy it and tick it off when it's done, rather than thinking of all the demands facing you. That way you're facing small waves rather than a tsunami. Mindfulness meditation is useful for this and a number of courses exist, increasingly aimed at health workers.
   - *Being assertive.* You need to realise you are in charge of your own destiny and not allow yourself to be tossed about by whatever comes your way. We all have to say no sometimes, whether inside work or in our private lives. Learning to challenge the thoughts that make you feel guilty about

saying no is essential if we are to avoid being overwhelmed by demands. The cognitive strategies in earlier chapters should help with guilt, but it's useful too to read a book on assertiveness, or get some coaching.

- *The compact.* One way of making sense of demands is to put them in the context of what is fair and reasonable. Are you being asked to do a great deal more than you deem acceptable? You can check this out with others, seeking advice both from those in your sort of job and from complete outsiders. You can also think about the types of agreements that exist, either explicitly, or implicitly, such as: 'You will work hard, with long hours and we will pay you well'; 'You will study and take exams for 10–15 years and we will give you a job for life, with a pension'; 'You will deal with suffering, death and uncertainty and we will reward you with status'. These sorts of agreements can be described as a 'compact' between doctors and the societies they live in, when the beliefs and assumptions about the job go beyond the job description. How this compact works[1] out will greatly influence how you feel about the demands placed upon you.
- *Value your patients.* It's all too easy to see patients as the 'enemy' yet they are why you are in medicine. Remember the more you invest in connecting with and caring for patients, the more you will get out of work. The idea of vocation has many benefits, as long as it's not used as a stick to beat you with; for example, 'You must see all these extra patients because it's your duty to'.

3 **Time management and delegation.** There are dozens of books on ways to manage your time better, and some are listed in the bibliography. Primarily time management involves making a list of what needs to be done; cutting out anything not essential (unless it's pleasure in which case you put it in a separate list); prioritising what's left; seeing whom you can delegate any of the tasks to; and getting on with it, using some of the strategies described above. In terms of Myers Brigg types, people who are Ps can find 101 ways of distracting themselves from what needs to be done next, so recognise that in yourself and put aside distractions till later. But it does matter that you have pleasure in your life and that some of this exists outside of the workplace, so don't rule out all of that. However, there will inevitably be times when you have to forgo something that you've planned, and sometimes you'll feel less stressed if you do that. It should be a rare event so, if it's happening a lot, then you need to think again about the demands that are on you and how to balance them better between work and the rest of your life. A friend or a coach might help here.

---

[1] See https://www.virginiamason.org/home/workfiles/HR/PhysicianCompact.pdf for an example of a compact in medicine.

Delegation can help too. Basically you need to delegate whenever there is someone below you with more skills than you, who could do it better or quicker, or who needs the training or a new challenge. Don't delegate tasks you don't like; be clear about what is to be done, check they've understood and acknowledge their achievements. Perfectionists (see Chapter 2) find delegation much more difficult which adds to their pressures, so do seek help with this if you feel the cap fits.

4. **Work with others.** Increasingly it is important to work effectively in teams. By working well with others, within medicine and in other professions, you will learn a range of skills and share the demands and get support in dealing with difficult issues. You won't like everyone you work with, but remember that holding strong resentments uses up valuable energy (and sleep) that could be used more pleasantly and productively.
5. **Remember your career anchor.** Each of us has one particular aspect of our work that we especially value and need to experience on a regular basis. For you this might be consulting with patients, clinical teaching, doing research, or using your hands in a surgical specialty. When this career anchor is absent or diminished, you will become dissatisfied, so it is important to discover your anchor and make sure you find it in your regular working week.
6. **Maintain your professional practice.** Take seriously your engagement with clinical medicine and the need to keep learning and developing. Processes for appraisal and revalidation may seem daunting (and irritating) but offer the chance to demonstrate the reflective learning you are doing. By keeping on top of the subject, you will enjoy your work more and feel better able to contribute to the care of patients and society in general.
7. **Consider different ways of working.** There will be times, both for men and women, when you might feel that part-time work will be best for you. Talk with your partners, friends and employers about this before you make a decision, but it can be really useful at different times of your life. It would be good to think parenting is shared equally between couples, but in reality this usually falls on women. Remember from Chapter 2 that women with children working full time in hospital medicine have by far the highest stress and depression levels so if you are in that group it becomes especially important to recognise when things are going wrong and to take action to change things. Whichever sex you are, if you have children, think about the possibility of part-time working or even a career break – a year to travel with them perhaps. It may be the only chance you ever have to really get to know them and it will be valuable for all of you.
8. **You might also think about a portfolio career.** Although many enjoy a working week entirely focused on one way of working in one geographical location, others (especially those who are Ns in Myers Briggs terms) benefit

from greater variety, especially as they get older. You may want to embrace a portfolio career which includes clinical work, managerial activity, clinical leadership or a more formal teaching role. For GPs this can involve working as a police or prison doctor, being a GP Trainer or GP Tutor, or being a GP with a Special Clinical Interest, in addition to mainstream general practice. Remember, though, that the more complex a career, the greater the difficulty when things go wrong. At certain times in your life you just have to be ruthless with yourself and cut out one or more of your range of activities.

9 **Ensure you have good management provision.** This applies particularly to general practice, where partnerships appoint practice managers who can control and guide management within their organisations. For others, it is important to engage constructively with managers, as usually their ultimate agendas and yours ought to be similar, if not identical. Clarify and confirm your compact with your employer as a way to make progress and feel fully connected to your place of work.

10.2 Demands change

1 **Early career.** The first few years as a qualified doctor require flexibility and clarity. You are suddenly expected to know more than you think you do, are full of uncertainties, and have skills that are still in an early phase of development. Despite this, people look to you for advice and reassurance, and you must now start to make decisions about the care of patients and begin to take clinical responsibility. At times there will be a multiplication of demands, from a range of patients, nursing colleagues and other doctors, sometimes spread out across the hospital. Some patients, if not the majority, will be acutely ill and needing intensive medical input and support, and some will die whilst under your care. At the same time, your social and domestic life will be in a state of transition. You may have moved away from close friends and peer group to take up a hospital job or rotation far away from your place of medical school training. You may have a partner who now is at a distance from you, or doing a medical job with a different rota pattern. To maintain proper contact with friends and family is demanding, not least of time and energy, especially where there are long distances to travel. You may feel this is putting a great deal of strain on your special relationships. Keeping in touch with people who matter is vital and is easier now, using phone, text, or e-mail, but we need face-to-face friends as well. The reduction in working hours in Europe and some other countries should allow more time for socialising or being with your partner. However, when at work, the pressure will often be extreme, so it's very important to use the time off duty also to recharge the physical, mental and emotional batteries.

> *Fiona was in her second postgraduate year, working in a busy medical unit, with a young doctor below her, and a registrar and consultant above her. She had moved away from her immediate social network to take up her rotation. She also had a widowed mother who suffered from bouts of clinical depression. Fiona struggled to cope when her mother is unwell. Recently Fiona had problems with a series of locum registrars who failed to follow local protocols and support her properly. Fortunately she was able to share her concerns with her consultant, and other team members also proved supportive when she asked them. They set up a daily handover session and rewrote the clinical protocols more clearly. She found a painting class and, even though she couldn't always turn up, she made new friends. She worked out a system to phone her mother at set times and set boundaries for visiting her. This allowed Fiona to feel more in control. She joined the local sports club and enjoyed getting physically fitter.*

Just like Fiona, you too will need to find ways of managing the complexity of your work and personal lives. The wise decision is to seek support and advice from others and to do something you enjoy outside of medicine. Ultimately it's you who must take or regain control, but others can help you do this.

2 **Mid-career.** Doctors in mid-career face a variety of competing demands and pressures. Now postgraduate training has passed, you are facing the greater challenge of being responsible to direct an area of clinical work. You will be part of a team, but its leadership and direction will increasingly be your task. It is likely you will be called to be a manager, as well as a clinician and leader, and new skills have to be developed, so don't miss a chance to go on relevant management courses. This is a period when hours can be long, and responsibilities to research, teaching and management, as well as clinical work, can overwhelm. New consultants have particularly high stress levels, probably with the leap in responsibility. It's definitely a time to get extra support from a mentor, especially as family concerns often become greater, with ageing parents, growing children and domestic partners wanting more of your time and engagement. Perhaps this is the time for a career break? Or perhaps you can find a few others in similar situations and form a group to meet monthly, offer support and other perspectives on difficulties, and just have a laugh. Doctors who have done this, in primary or in secondary care, say that they find it enormously helpful.

   Financial pressures may also intrude and you would be wise to review the sorts of expenditure you will be facing before taking on too many financial outgoings, as these can become burdensome and an extra set of demands. There is considerable evidence that happiness does not always increase with wealth!

Kumar had been a medical partner in a large, busy GP practice for five years. He was thinking of becoming a GP Trainer and developing a special interest in minor surgery. At the same time he found his expertise in business and management meant that the practice manager and senior partner required his help to run the practice organisation. With a growing family he felt he needed to buy a larger house, and he worried about finding schools for his children, thinking he may have to pay to go privately. He found he spent longer at work with so much to do, and saw less of the family.

Following conversations with his mentor, Kumar was able to negotiate to spend one session per week on the business side of the practice, as well as delegate some smaller tasks to a colleague. He decided to continue in GP training, but put the minor surgery interest to one side for the present. Having reviewed his time management, he stopped interruptions whilst consulting, which freed up time and made him more efficient. His work flowed better, and he was now usually home on time. With financial advice, he began to organise his retirement pensions and put the purchase of a new house on hold.

Kumar's story highlights a range of issues that can build up without realising it – taking on more tasks (without dropping others), developing wider professional roles such as teaching, and being sucked into the need to do more to increase income – a good time to say 'Enough'! His compact with his practice partnership has allowed a redefining of his role to take up a more formal position as executive partner. The use of a mentor, a clarification of your priorities, a modified work plan, increased delegation and a time management review will allow you to cope better.

3 **Late career.** As you get older the demands of seniority become more pronounced. It is no longer possible to claim that you are too junior or inexperienced to take a leading role. Managers will come to you for solutions, and you will go to them to help sort out the big concerns of your department or area of work. You will still need to keep up to date with the medical literature, as well as be involved in teaching and research. You are aware that your clinical performance, as well as your physical stamina, will at some point drop off. Yet you must still fulfil the requirements of appraisal and continuing professional development targets and deliver high quality patient care.

If you've not already done it, you will be planning how to manage your retirement income, ideally getting specialist financial advice for this. Preparing for retirement is something you would be wise to do, not least in working out how to make the transition from working life to retirement. A career in medicine allows this to be a gradual process if desired, with a shift to part-time working, or the ability to maintain certain areas of work such as medico-legal and private work.

Older doctors sometimes find their clinical work is less satisfying, and it's a good time to develop your role as mentor to others, and to begin writing or painting or any pastime that can be enjoyed in retirement too. Think about what you dreamt of doing and find ways to do some part of it at least. Late career is a time too when new ideas can be tried out and exciting possibilities adopted. The future is never certain, so best to make the most of the time.

Bill was a senior consultant in neurology. He ran the regional service for epilepsy, whilst also directing clinical neurology services in his hospital. He maintained a research interest, as well as having teaching duties and facilitating various clinical meetings at local, national and international level. Increasingly he was feeling weighed down by the demands at work, as well as struggling to maintain his social friendships.

Through using a personal coach Bill clarified his key work objectives and personal goals. He learnt to be more assertive in his management role, and reduce his exposure to travel demands by limiting the scope of his wider professional roles. He engaged a financial advisor to work with him on pension planning and took out a gym subscription to improve his general wellbeing.

Bill has made the active move to find and then work with a life coach. This has allowed him to review his priorities and focus his attention on what he wants for the final years of his career and what he wants to begin to develop as he moves towards retirement. We could do this alone or with friends, but it's often much easier to have an independent person point out aspects of you and your life that have become so commonplace to you that they are easily overlooked.

In conclusion, demands need to be tackled regularly and differently at every stage of your career so that you feel you are maintaining some control over your work, and have sufficient time in your private life to enjoy yourself and those close to you.

Bibliography

Allan D. *Getting Things Done: How to Achieve Stress-Free Productivity*. 2002, Piatkus, London.

Evans C. *Time Management for Dummies*. 2008, John Wiley, Chichester.

Handy C. *The Age of Unreason: New Thinking for a New World*. 2002, Random House, London.

Chapter 11 **Can you afford emotions?**

Medical teaching has traditionally been pretty clear in its teaching about the need to suppress emotional reactions in dealings with your patients. Whereas the rules of good practice for nursing usually mention the word 'compassion' this is not the case for medicine. The traditional line was always to maintain 'professional detachment' – polite but with a very clear boundary: kept in place by the secure knowledge that 'I'm the doctor and you're the patient'. This helps you to carry out intimate and painful procedures or give distressing news without getting too involved. Indeed, doctors would be specifically advised against showing their feelings, particularly in relation to death and dying. A doctor who shed a tear would be viewed as a risk to the efficient running of the department. The need for you to remain distant and unemotional remains the norm in most countries, but current teaching methods are to some extent breaking this rule down.

This chapter considers the role of compassion in health care, and what blocking it or allowing it might mean to you and your patients. Here the boxed stories are in the first person, whether from doctors or from patients. This is because compassion is a felt experience – an emotion felt by the patient and by the doctor – so stories have to come from them. It's clear from the patients' accounts that they want something that shows the doctor cares about them as a fellow suffering human being. It's clear too that if you want to be remembered for good things rather than for bad – since both kind actions and cruel ones are remembered vividly – then paying attention to the emotional side of medicine matters a lot.

I was 10 weeks pregnant when I began to bleed a little. I went up to the hospital, by then doubled up with pain. Three young doctors came into the cubicle, two men and a woman. When they saw I was unmarried one asked me what I had done to get rid of the baby. I told them I wanted the baby, was living happily with the father and planned to marry

---

next month. Two of them ignored this, gave me an internal despite my pain. They never looked at me, just at my abdomen, and talked to each other and just shrugged when everything was clear. The third doctor, from Africa, held my eyes and held my hand. He called me by my name and looked ashamed. When the two had gone, chatting away between themselves, he explained what they'd been doing. Later, when I lost the baby, he came to the ward to say he was sorry. I won't forget them ever, but even more I won't forget his kindness. It was a long time ago and I hope things have changed.

Things have changed. Nowadays within undergraduate and early postgraduate training more emphasis is placed on psychosocial skills, including teaching politeness and improving rapport with patients or discussing issues like compassion and empathy within an ethics course. This is a good thing, of course, but it's still not regarded as 'core'; students and young doctors report that these subjects are viewed as somewhat irrelevant because they see an emphasis on clinical teaching as the thing that matters most, both academically and clinically. One young doctor told us:

It's part of what is seen as soft and fluffy. People ask 'Is it on the exam?' and of course it isn't so it's hard to see it as important. Where it is judged, it's like a tick-box exercise – a mark for shaking hands, for saying your name …

In a study that asked students how they learnt about empathy,[1] one student wrote: ' … *with every test score posted … it was a constant reminder that competition and personal gain were the essence of medical school. Knowledge to succeed in medical school was the 'end all', not knowledge to help people battle diseases and decrease suffering.*'

However you felt about these things when you first came into medicine, however naturally compassionate you were, the biomedical model still rules within medical training and other aspects of care tend to fade away rather than balancing it. In fact, despite the growing emphasis on the psychosocial model, in many studies from around the world empathy has been shown to reduce steadily throughout medical training. Good as it is in many ways, one significant problem with the biomedical model is that its scientific basis tends to make the patient simply an object to be studied, which of course helps you to maintain your distance and not get too involved. But that doesn't always feel good as the two accounts here show.

---

[1]Wear, Zarconi. Can compassion be taught? Let's ask our students. *J Gen Int Med* 2008;**23**:948–53.

> *We were looking after an elderly patient who was sitting up in bed, bag packed, because he'd been told he was able to go home. We were all scared of this consultant – she was big on science but poor on compassion. I had presented the patient to her, along with our plan of discharge. She didn't really look at him or introduce herself. Just read the notes and then said he would not go home as he needed further tests. The consultant then just walked away and I had to follow because she was outlining the tests, although I wanted to go back and explain to the patient who was devastated and clearly trying not to cry. I felt ghastly and ashamed of being part of it all.*
>
> *We were on a round in a female gynae ward and the surgeon would talk to us all rather than the patient, and then turn to her and say 'Don't worry; we'll take it out for you'. This happened a few times, which was ghastly enough. But then we came to a woman who was reading the Guardian. He talked to her throughout, answered her questions, explained the procedure, checked she understood. When we left he looked at us proudly: 'Never trust a Guardian reader', he said. 'They're the ones who sue'. A few people tittered, but I think they felt embarrassed more than anything. I just felt dreadful. I hope I never end up like that.*

Good role models are a wonderful gift, both to model yourself on, and to support you. They will help you to maintain the compassion you have left, or even regain it fully but, as these stories make clear, there are still plenty of poor role models and they often hold power and status that can seem pretty attractive. Now nurses too have turned their profession into degree courses; their broader caring function has somewhat faded, and they often face disillusionment at the distance between what they expected of themselves and the health service, and the reality they face. Patients everywhere are asking 'Where has the humanity gone?'

What makes all this more difficult are the changes in the health service outlined in Chapter 1 – the turnover of beds, the demise of the firm, shift-systems, more complaints and litigation, and more seriously ill patients which sometimes mean less chance to get to know them.

11.1 Is compassion good for you?

This is a tricky one. Compassion – that human quality of understanding suffering in others and wanting to do something about it – is a core part of every great religion in the world, particularly Buddhism, and it's certainly good for the patients: it actually makes a difference to many aspects of their experience and even their recovery. They want to know that the doctor understands and is treating them as fellow humans as well as patients. They want the generosity that is involved in real dialogue as opposed to simple factual information (though that's good too), and recognition of the man or woman they were rather than only the sick or dying person they have become. And they want kindness: those little gestures that indicate you're understanding their distress and doing what you can to relieve it. But is that good for you too? We have to say, it depends.

First of all, compassion is a normal human emotion, though it doesn't come ready-formed, but grows over a lifetime. It is also probably adaptive in an evolutionary sense. People (in fact, mammals in general) want caring behaviours – they need to be stroked, held, hear the right voice tone and facial expression since these actions stimulate neurohormones such as oxytocin and opiates which have a calming effect, alter pain thresholds and the immune and digestive systems. Because we want this, we probably have to give it too – that's what is adaptive and so normal about giving compassion. In fact, studies show that those with higher empathy actually have lower stress and burnout levels, so chances are being good to others can be good for you.

But evolution isn't always neat. It's likely that these benefits will depend on your relationship with the person: it's very easy to be kind and empathic with your child or your best friend, and probably easier to feel something for patients who are close to you in some way than it is with others who seem very different – the drug addicts, the obese, the elderly, the insane. These are the 'it's their own fault' patients, or the difficult or different ones. With the increased severity of illness for in-patients, and the rise in obesity and drug use, more and more patients fall into these categories. It's always difficult to treat these people as equals, to have a real dialogue with them human-to-human.

Moreover, there is a very inconvenient conflicting drive – again probably evolutionary – to stay away from disease and death as much as you can. This is because (a) you might catch it, and (b) where one person dies, others often do, whether from an enemy or from illness. You might also want to stay away from distress, because studies have shown that viewing another person's distress actually lowers your own pain threshold. In fact, this empathic response is so strong that, if you are causing pain to some part of another person's body, the same part of your own body will often feel at least a twinge, if not worse. In addition, if you make a mistake over a patient – and who doesn't do that from time to time – then your empathy levels towards that patient reduce!

Alongside these various barriers to compassion there is also the fact that the suffering or death of another brings home our own vulnerability and mortality. Rather than recognising that it is just those two conditions that we all share in common, it is often less scarey to be able to put ourselves on one side of the barrier with 'the healthy' and the patients on the other side with 'disease'.

So there are a number of reasons why you might decide that allowing feelings of compassion towards your patients is potentially too distressing, especially as you've been taught something about keeping your boundaries. Of course you must keep the boundary in terms of finance or sex, but buttoning down the emotional hatches is done at a cost to you, as John's story shows.

I was a very traditional problem-focussed scientist in the way I practised medicine but, looking back, I always knew something was always missing. I felt guilty about not using my humanity and yet I didn't want to drop down any of the barriers. Most of my colleagues worked in the same way. My teenage son got ill and was left in severe pain for nearly an hour while people phaffed around, even though my complaints got so loud. And we were treated all the time like objects, irritations even. His few days in hospital were such an eye-opener to me. I knew now what it was like to be ignored, to be treated as a non-person without kindness from either nurses or doctors. Horrible. I started thinking about my own practice, the way I blocked out feeling and generosity to patients. At the suggestion of a friend I found a course on mindfulness meditation, and things began to change for me. I stopped being a clinical director because that was getting in the way and now I just treat patients and love it. Now I enjoy talking with them and I've never felt so fulfilled by medicine.

11.2 Using dialogue

One way to be compassionate but not to be overwhelmed or merged with another person is to talk to them human-to-human, using dialogue. Good communication of information is important, but dialogue goes further. It's not doctor to patient, but two interested people having a conversation. It's about:

- appreciating the differences between you and so keeping the boundary there;
- talking to the real person, not reacting to a stereotype;
- talking human-to-human, not clinician to patient, with a language of participation;
- recognising who they are now, but also who and what they were before they became ill;
- and being aware of what your actions or attitudes will mean for them.

The account in the first box in this chapter and in the carer's story that follows illustrates how simply it is done and what a difference it makes.

The afternoon we arrived at the hospice a doctor and nurse came to talk to us. My husband was terminally ill, looked like a skeleton, and had just been discharged from three dreadful weeks in hospital where he'd been given painful procedures without us quite understanding why, had been left for an hour in excruciating pain, and had been starved for days on end because he dropped off the list day after day. He was so much worse now so a hospice was suggested and we'd gone there reluctantly just to get his medication right. I could see he wasn't going to be very welcoming to another doctor at this stage. But she asked about him, not about his illness: what had he done for work, what did he enjoy now, what did we do together. Gradually he seemed to grow back into the large, active, witty man he'd been. She spent all the time he needed, she answered his questions honestly, she allowed silence, and she addressed the whole man – the one he was as well as the one he had become. It was a generous, kind and honest conversation with lots of laughter as he entertained her. He stayed there peacefully till he died.

A remark early on in your dialogue that tries to understand what patients or carers might be feeling will let them know straight away that you're interested and that they can talk to you more easily than they might expect; for example: 'I guess this is a bit scarey'; or 'You must have thought I'd never get to you'; or 'I know this is an awful lot to take in'; 'pretty exhausting for you, all this?'. In addition, you can get them to talk to you more equally by asking some getting-to-know-you questions such as:

- What do/did you enjoy most about your work/leisure?
- Who will be affected by your illness?
- What concerns you most?
- What should I know about you that will let me take good care of you – likes? dislikes? fears?

This is how you would talk to someone you've just met of your own age, class, health and intelligence; it's really no different to that.

11.3 Your health too

But this is not a book about how to be good to patients; it's about how to be good to yourself. What we are saying is that you will feel much better about yourself if you know you have been kind and caring to your patients as well as helped them clinically. Kindness might nowadays seem to be limited to people like Mother Theresa or Nelson Mandela, but that's not true: we all have it naturally and it always makes us feel better afterwards.

However, you will find it less easy to be compassionate to others if you are not kind to yourself. If you constantly find you compare yourself unfavourably to your peers; if you are unduly self-critical; if you bully yourself with words like 'loser', 'not good enough', 'unlovable', 'weak', 'outsider' – then you will not only feel depressed, you'll also find it very difficult to be kind to patients. It would be good to think that a flow of compassion went right through the hospital or surgery, so that your colleagues or seniors were so kind to you that you found it easy to be good to your patients. But we know that isn't always so and, if you wait till it happens, you might be disappointed never to feel warm in the glow of their appreciation. You need instead to challenge your own thoughts about yourself; to correct yourself when you think self-critical words or worries like those above. Tell yourself it's just your internal bully, and consult the list you have of all the good things you are and you have done. Failing at one thing doesn't make a person a failure; making one small error with a patient has to be judged in the light of all the good that you've done: you don't need to punish yourself nor your patient! You'll know when you've been less kind than you could, but you will also register the times when your kindness made a difference.

Stress makes it harder to show compassion, so addressing this is very important (see Chapters 5 and 6). But in addition try to join or develop a group of peers or others who can talk about the difficult and upsetting events that happen in medicine. In the States, and now beginning in England and Australia, are Schwarz seminars – voluntary multi-disciplinary groups of health workers who use a monthly meeting to discuss painful and difficult encounters with patients and carers. Balint groups used to exist in general practice with a similar function, but restricted just to doctors. What the members do is express their distress and uncertainty – did they do the right thing and how difficult it had been. This might seem to heap one stress on top of another, but research over two decades has shown that talking about distressing events, big and small, has a beneficial effect not only on our mental health but even on our immune system, on rheumatoid arthritis, eczema and other conditions. As we've said before, talking about it is powerful, not just a passive activity. And the research also shows that, if you can't find anyone to talk to about these things, then write about it. That is almost as good.

The other way to help you to show your natural kindness and to dare to feel emotions is through mindfulness training. This is a form of meditation which is being used increasingly, and particularly for health workers. It's regarded as good for patients and staff alike. Like speaking about traumas or upsets, it too enhances antibody production and other immune system responses, but also increases self-compassion which in turn affects positively life satisfaction while reducing stress, depression, burnout and anxiety.

In answer to the question in the title of the chapter, you can afford to allow yourself to feel for your patients, but you need to feel good about yourself and you need the support of colleagues and friends in order to do it. All these methods – working on your negative thoughts, talking about your difficulties, writing about them, learning mindfulness meditation – will help you to practise medicine the way you wanted to when you first entered it. They will put you back in touch with your humanity, let you feel good about yourself and make you a much better doctor.

Bibliography

Chochinov H. Dignity and the essence of medicine: the A, B, C, and D of dignity conserving care. *BMJ* 2007;**335**:184–7.

Firth-Cozens J, Cornwell J. *Enabling Compassion in Acute Services*. 2009, The King's Fund: http://www.kingsfund.org.uk/research/projects/the_point_of_care_improving_patients_experience/compassion/the_point_of_care_.html

Førde R, Aasland OG. Moral distress among Norwegian doctors. *J Med Ethics* 2008;**34**:5221–5.

Frank AW. *The Renewal of Generosity: Illness, Medicine and How to Live*. 2004, University of Chicago Press, London & Chicago.

Chapter 12 **To err is human**

Doctors, being human, have always made mistakes, and these can be just as devastating as when the signalman on the railway line pressed the wrong button, or the airline pilot fell asleep, or the bus driver put the double-decker into reverse instead of first gear as he waited at the lights on the hill. Now we have started counting health care errors around the world, we find that, whether we're a patient or a doctor, the numbers are frighteningly at high. Frightening for patients and for doctors. Studies in the UK and several other countries have shown that 8–12% of patients admitted to hospital are harmed by the treatment they receive; about half of this is preventable. Many of the problems are quite minor, but a proportion involve serious disability or the death of a patient. And in a more recent study over a third of the young doctors participating reported at least one major error during the three months of the study period. As these studies used self-reported errors or ones recorded in the notes, chances are the figure is conservative. Studies show that most doctors find making a serious error extremely upsetting, and sometimes their distress over what happened lasts for years, especially if they have never felt able to talk to anyone about it.

Most occupations develop systems to attempt to cancel out the inevitable errors that humans make, but there will always be times when something uniquely human and unexpected sweeps through the system and causes a catastrophe. Professor James Reason demonstrated the causes of mistakes with his three-buckets diagram, the buckets usually being filled with an unpleasantly brown substance.

The system, designed to stop error happening in any industry or profession, is made up of the three buckets: it needs to address the characteristics of the task in terms of the dangers it presents; the varying contexts that might

---

How to Survive in Medicine. By © Jenny Firth-Cozens. Published 2010 Blackwell Publishing.

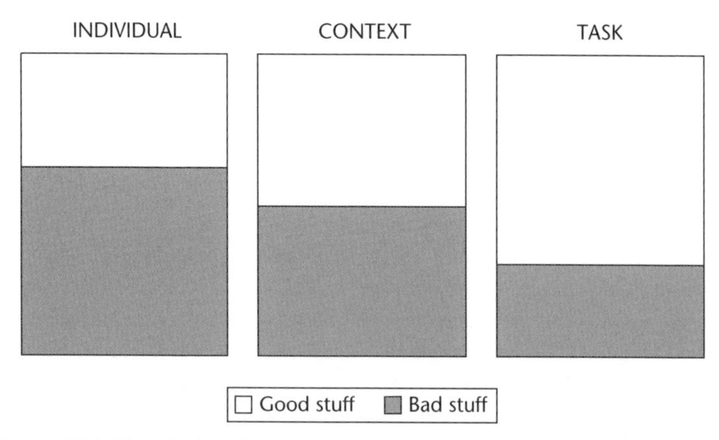

Figure 12.1 Three-buckets diagram.

make those dangers greater or less; and the individuals doing the task, with their own competences, personalities, stress levels and so on. In most industries, such as aviation or railways, individuals are less important and most of their potential errors can be over-ruled by safety elements embedded in the system. In health care too, the system is often the problem that underlies harm that might occur to a patient for example, poorly designed infusion pumps or having to work with six different pumps in a single hospital invites error no matter now conscientious you are. Nevertheless, the individual remains a very important aspect of the quality of care, far more so than in other industries. In some specialties, such as surgery or anaesthetics, this importance is reduced considerably by the public nature of the task and the vigilance of the team. In others, such as general practice or psychiatry, the interaction is very much more private and the individual becomes even more key to the outcome.

So, in this chapter, we are going to look at some of the things which might lead you to making an error, and what to do if this happens.

12.1 Risk and the individual

1 **Competence.** Inexperience is going to be a factor in all doctors at some point, whether you are just out of medical school or struggling to learn a new skill much later in your career. With good supervision and appropriate ways to gain experience, this should not be problematic. Once done, however, competence is still bound to vary. We all have different physical and intellectual strengths and weaknesses which will lead to different

levels of skill for various tasks. Most of us recognise these, try to improve the areas where we are weak, but then design our careers around them if we feel they are not up to scratch. A few, however, push on regardless, sure that eventually that skill will be gained despite growing evidence to the contrary.

In both these scenarios the most important thing is to get feedback as early as possible. First, it's essential that you don't give up a potentially fruitful career because you have not yet developed the relevant skill or you've made a single error. So discuss your doubts and difficulties with someone more experienced, an educational supervisor, a mentor and with colleagues too if you feel able. The more feedback you can get before giving up, the better the choice will be. On the other hand, you need feedback even more if your confidence levels are very high and you feel that you will manage to conquer that skill in the end. Too much confidence – especially if it slips into arrogance – is a dangerous trait in medicine. What's more, the less skilled we are in a particular task, the less insight we have into this. Paradoxically, as you start to gain the skills, your estimation of competence reduces!

2 **Personality.** Research into the disposition of doctors whose professional performance is often questionable is in its infancy, but the variety of studies that exist consistently show that there are some enduring aspects of personality which do influence the way these doctors approach safety and other aspects of quality. For example, there is gathering evidence that those who are disciplined by US medical-licensing boards are more likely than controls to have shown some aspect of unprofessional behaviour at medical school, whether it was alcohol or drug-related or behaving inappropriately with a patient, showing rage, and so on.

Some people can see the risk in situations more easily than others and this is likely to affect patient safety unless it's taken into account. One surgeon we know uses his early morning swim as a time to think about his cases that day and of all the possible things that he could anticipate going wrong. This ability to anticipate risk has been linked to better outcomes and can undoubtedly be done by most people with practice. But some of those who can see the risk still do dangerous things: the well-documented 'risky personality' has only rarely been considered in health care, but has been studied widely elsewhere and found to influence a range of safety behaviours. This personality type is more likely to take part in various sensation-seeking activities from excessive alcohol to extreme sports, and sometimes to show very disinhibited behaviours. While specialties such as surgery demand that doctors are bound to take some risks, it is really important that anyone who feels and enjoys the buzz that taking a risk can produce receives regular feedback from team members rather than acting unilaterally most of the time.

3 **Health.** There are numerous physical illnesses which are likely to increase your chances of error or at least to make you work less well. For example, doctors with Parkinson's disease, multiple sclerosis, arthritis or even diabetes need to work closely with occupational health to make sure they are not exceeding their capabilities. This is important for the patient, of course, but also for them. Needless to say, all the dementias are likely to create problems even in the early days, but it is vital too to have a thorough psycho-neurological examination when you have had any sort of head injury: even relatively mild ones can cause behavioural and cognitive changes, usually temporarily.

Doctors with mental illnesses such as bipolar disorder have a very difficult time in medicine, often facing stigma and real difficulties in managing their illness while performing such a stressful job (see Chapter 4 on career choice). One young doctor with bipolar disorder reported:

> *As a part timer, in one A&E job I was getting my rota only a week in advance – which had a massive affect on my personal and social life. This led to social isolation and eventually contributed, along with the rotation difficulties, to me being hospitalized.*

While disability discrimination legislation may say that reasonable adjustments have to be made for these doctors, the definition of reasonable is difficult to decide and doctors often prefer to keep their illness secret while they can. However, this can be very dangerous because they may need adjustments to their working day so that there is some consistency and they are not ending up exhausted and ill. They are much better served by using honesty in supervision and appraisal and finding someone to mentor them through difficult times. Sometimes this can lead to better care for you, and much less risk to your patients; for example:

> *I had regular OH assessments. They paid for a private psychiatric assessment and created a role specifically for me, fitting me onto the rota so I had a role in my own right. I received regular mentoring with my supervising consultant, and removal of on-call as and when necessary. People were great.*

4 **Stress and depression.** Error, stress and depression are intimately linked. Not only are you more likely to make errors when your stress levels are high or when you're feeling depressed, but also it seems the making of the error goes on to make you more burnt out, stressed and less empathic, and leads to an even greater chance of making more errors in the next few months.

For the sake of patients, of your career, and of your health and wellbeing *do* something about your stress or depression (see Chapters 5 and 6) and talk to someone about the error you made. If you don't, then its effects will stay with you and cause various problems not only in terms of future stress and errors, but also possibly shifts in your career path as you re-align it to try to avoid such situations in the future. People learn from their errors, but they can learn inappropriate things as well as good ones, and the only way to ensure that the mistake you made ends up making you a better doctor is to admit to it to someone who will help you to learn well from it.

5 **Exhaustion.** Most studies find a significant deterioration with sleep deprivation, in particular with concentration and reaction time. A study of surgical house officers[1] found that, following a weekend on-call, significant impairment took place in concentration and speed, and they were less confident and happy and more confused. Impaired performance in general was highly negatively related (–0.5 to –0.6) to the number of hours of sleep. They estimate that, in terms of magnitude, the impairment to vigilance was close to that caused by 0.7 g/kg alcohol which, as they point out, is close to the legal limit in the UK. There is evidence too from military studies that individual errors increase with fatigue. However, over time it seems that the team can compensate for these errors, so those who worked together over a longer period may have higher individual error scores but lower team error scores than those working together only briefly. These studies measure extremely long shifts and it may be that it's not so much the number of hours you work as the amount of sleep you get which causes the decline in performance, as the quote from this senior doctor illustrates:

> *When I was working as a principal in general practice I was on call every fourth night and frequently had to do night visits. I became so tired it became more and more difficult to motivate myself to get out of bed when patients phoned. One lady phoned me at 2 am to say her husband couldn't sleep. I nearly hit the roof as I knew she'd been calling my partners with the same thing. I gave advice over the phone. Several days later her husband died; he had an ischemic leg which had been causing pain and interrupting his sleep. None of us had realized what was going on because we all got so irritated by his wife that we didn't stay long enough to examine him properly. If we had been fresh and more patient, this could not have happened.*

Working and sleeping hours are inevitably related and ending extended work shifts in some places has led to better sleep and fewer cognitive failures: most doctors, it seems, use their shorter working hours to get more sleep rather than partying longer.

---

[1]Wesnes K, Walker M, Walker L. Cognitive performance and mood after a weekend on-call in a surgical unit. *Br J Surg* 1997;**84**:493–5.

12.2 When an error happens

Serious mistakes are devastating for doctors of all ages. When asked to look back at important events throughout their careers, doctors will most often describe an error they made. Naturally there is no evidence to show that it feels worse when you try to bury an error compared to when you admit one, but this is likely to be the case since trying to cope with an upsetting event or trauma by self-denial or by trying to avoid thinking about it actually makes the effects continue longer.

Over the last 10 years, around the world, health services have attempted to improve patient safety by getting medical and nursing staff to admit their mistakes or to report those of others. In this way it was thought that major systems problems could be recognised and addressed, and organisations such as the UK National Patient Safety Agency began to do this through anonymous reporting. However, the aim to make organisational cultures more open and trustworthy so that people can report more freely knowing they were unlikely to face blame has by no means materialised.

So what should you do? Medical regulators around the world have emphasised that individual doctors must take responsibility not only for ensuring their own medical performance, but also that of their peers and superiors. Indeed, a recent BMA study of UK doctors qualifying in 2006 stated that 96.3% of those questioned agreed that they were responsible not only for their own actions but also corporately for the action of medical colleagues. This figure had been 83.5% for those qualifying in 1995 when asked at the same stage of their careers.

> Pete had become aware that some of his dermatology colleagues were failing to send all skin specimens to the laboratory for histological analysis. He brought this up with one of them, who said that it wasn't necessary to send every tiny bit of tissue or cauterised fragment. Pete disagreed. He could have left the issue there on the basis that he had raised the concern and thereby fulfilled his obligation. Yet he remained unhappy and so brought up the matter again at the departmental meeting. After further discussion, Pete's view was accepted, even though some had been irritated by the proposal.

12.3 That was close!

Reporting near-misses – where you almost made an error and why – would be just as helpful as reporting actual errors and would mean that staff would then not run the risk of losing their jobs because they reported their own mishaps or those of others. However, this reporting almost never happens. We humans are basically an over-optimistic species and, instead of learning from our near-misses, we tend to ignore them as if they didn't occur. For example, when Hurricane Hugo hit and devastated a small prairie town, that town rebuilt itself with every sort of protective building strategy available. The town five miles away, which had so narrowly escaped its ravages, did nothing at all. It takes real concentration and teamwork to recognise and learn from near-misses, but it's the most worthwhile exercise you can do as a team, so make the effort whenever you can. (Chapter 13 considers ways for senior doctors to manage patient safety.)

12.4 Complaints and litigation

Most health care staff want to do a very good job and so find it very distressing to do something wrong which results in a patient suffering more than they have to, or even dying. However, in these situations it does not come as unexpected that the patient or relatives decide to complain or to make a legal claim. The blow is often much harder when doctors feel they have done a good or good-enough job with a patient, even provided optimal care, and still a complaint is made. So much of our self-image is tied up in what we do that, whether it goes on to a disciplinary body or not, the complaint feels like a personal attack on our very being.

Where complaints are taken further towards discipline, then the long drawn-out process is probably the most traumatic of a doctor's career and depression is very common. If you find yourself in this situation, organise some very good help early on – not just from friends because, if you start to have doubts about your ability, their insistence about how good you really are will begin to feel hollow. Much better to get yourself a mentor, counsellor or therapist right at the start of the process. The Medical Defence Societies offer sound advice and support, as can professional bodies such as your national or local medical association.

There is, however, good evidence that the way you discuss care and outcomes with a patient or the patient's relatives when they feel something has gone wrong will affect the likelihood of whether they complain or sue, or not. For example, findings show that apologies take away most of the anger and reduce the chance of litigation, although this response needs careful liaison with your employer, especially when done in writing. Where patients or relatives feel that their doctor or nurse has shown compassion, they are much less likely to be litigious: dialogue which shows you understand their frustration or suffering is good for both of you (see Chapter 11).

> Julia was aware that she should have visited the patient urgently at 3 a.m. rather than tell him to go to the emergency department at the local hospital. She should at least have organised ambulance transport. In the event the patient had survived a heart attack, but only just. Julia decided to come clean with the patient, arranging to see him and apologise. She did not try to defend her tiredness or confusion after being woken in the middle of the night. Julia also confirmed that the practice would review the case at a significant event audit meeting, seek to learn from the error, and put in place clear guidance for the future. Her honest apology, plus the commitment to do better in the future, won the patient over and he continued to see her as his doctor.

The reactions of patients and their carers are likely to be similar to those of your colleagues if they see you make an honest mistake. On the whole, you will find that staff support you well and do everything they can to minimise the effects of your error on the patient. By admitting it you are much more likely to be able to help others recognise and attend to the systems problems that might underlie it. In every sense it is important that you maintain good relationships at work, and evidence shows colleagues tend to help a doctor through errors if:

- It's a single mistake and the doctor is 'otherwise good'.
- The doctor says he or she is sorry.
- The doctor shows insight – appreciates the error has been made and so can work with others to ensure it doesn't happen again.

All over the world, women doctors are complained about less and face far less discipline and litigation than men do. It may be that they actually make fewer errors and behave better generally; certainly, there is evidence that they have superior communication skills. However, it may also be that they handle errors and complaints better, showing more emotional intelligence and compassion in their interactions.

You're not invincible and you're doing a very difficult job. If you make sure that on a daily basis you approach patients and colleagues without arrogance, human-to-human, giving and seeking help as necessary, then your reputation will help you through any errors you may make, and what you learn from the experience will make you a better doctor.

Bibliography

Cox J, et al. *Understanding Doctors' Performance*. 2005, Radcliffe Publishing, Abingdon.

Firth-Cozens J, Greenhalgh J. Doctors' perceptions of the links between stress and lowered clinical care. *Soc Sci Med* 1997;**44**:1017–22.

Firth-Cozens J. Doctors with difficulties: why so few women? *Postgrad Med J* 2008;**84**:318–320.

Hayes K, Thomas M. *Clinical Risk Management in Primary Care.* 2005, Radcliffe Publishing, Abingdon.

Kohatsu ND, Gould D, Ross LK, Fox PJ. Characteristics associated with physician discipline. *Arch Int Med* 2004;**164**:653–8.

Roter D, et al. Physician gender effects in medical communication. *JAMA* 2002;**288**:756–64.

Vincent CA. *Patient Safety*. 2006. Elsevier, Kidlington.

Vincent CA. Understanding and responding to adverse events. *New Eng J Med* 2003;**348**:1052–8.

Chapter 13 Managing the stress and problems of others

At least one in four of your team or your organisation is likely to be suffering above threshold levels of stress at any one time so the cost is tremendous: poor performance, absence, early retirement, litigation – even health and safety issues. It's worth doing something about stress, both for the individual and for the organisation. This chapter provides the doctor who manages others with some preventive strategies and ways to deal with the stressed or under-performing doctor. This is particularly important for patient safety, as we outlined in the Introduction, so in Figure 13.1 we show a systems diagram of the main causes and outcomes of stress in doctors and their relationship to patient care, sometimes direct and sometimes indirect. In the flow system at the bottom we list the interventions that can be made at various points. Some of these are primary or preventive interventions, focussing on the large organisational box on the left, and some are secondary, focussing there again, but also on the individual doctor.

13.1 Primary interventions

1 **Recognising the signs of stress.** Everybody suffers from stress at one time or another. The problem is in not recognising it and letting it continue so that it slips into something more serious and harder to change. So perhaps the most important intervention of all is to enable people to recognise their own stress and that of their colleagues. You can do this through leaflets, recommending books, posters, the intranet and by stress management workshops.
2 **Stress management workshops.** These need to teach people to recognise the feelings, thoughts and behaviours which might indicate their stress levels are rising (see Chapter 5) and then to provide some simple solutions for tackling this. Although it's only geared to preventing problems or helping

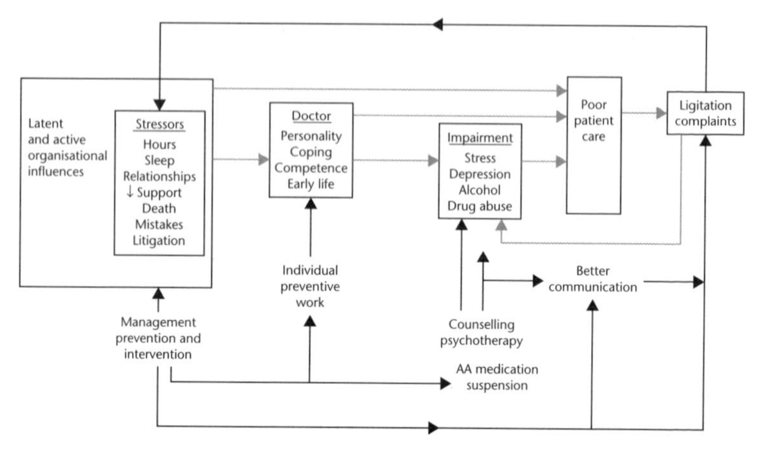

Figure 13.1 A systems approach to the causes of poor patient care. (Firth-Cozens J. Interventions to improve physicians' well-being and patient care. Soc Sci Med 2001;52:215–22.)

with transient stressors, for many participants a good workshop will go further than this and act as a spur to tackling longer-standing difficulties. Their benefits have been shown in a number of studies, but one that was directed at hospitals in a randomly controlled trial showed that the organisational intervention, which included a stress management workshop, resulted in a fall of annual malpractice claims from 31 to 9, while the control group of hospital remained virtually unchanged.

3 **Teams and team leadership.** It is particularly important that leaders can recognise stress in their staff, and know how to handle it well. In fact, if team leaders are taught leadership skills and how to manage their teams properly, the teams' stress levels will go down. Organisational psychologists have shown that the stress level of a team is an excellent indicator of the quality of that team in terms of all aspects of its work: members of good teams have lower stress levels and provide better care. The criteria of a good team were described in Chapter 1. Although most health service staff see themselves as working in teams, data from the UK's National Health Service staff surveys show that a large proportion of them work in 'pseudo-teams'; that is, the staff say they are in a team, but it does not meet the criteria. The fewer criteria that are met, the more those team members make errors and suffer harassment and violence, and the more their organisations show lower quality of care, worse use of resources and even, it is suggested, higher patient mortality.

---

[1]Jones JW, Barge BN, Steffy BD et al, Stress and medical malpractice: organisational risk assessment and intervention, 1988; J.Appl.Psychol, 4, 727-35.

The shift from uni-professional hospital teams, such as a medical firm or a nursing team, to multi-professional groups working within a clinical area to provide a service, demands new teamwork skills. One of the problems some consultants notice with this new way of working is that some young doctors no longer appear to have much commitment to their jobs, seem to regard them as very 9 to 5, and appear dissatisfied about far more than their predecessors, despite the much shorter hours and greater support. It may be that, rather than providing them only with all sorts of 'parental' help, such as educational tutors, mentors, etc. outside the team, we should make supportive relationships, whether tutors or their senior doctors, rather more two-way and adult so that responsibilities are emphasised as much as what you can do for them. When people have only a dependent, parent–child relationship, they tend to feel all sorts of old resentments as they did as adolescents. An emphasis on the compact, discussed in Chapter 10, will help to set a more meaningful way of managing young staff.

4 **Regular meetings.** One of the criteria of a good team is that it should meet regularly. This is important for patient safety, but it also matters for the stress and morale of its staff. Staff members must be given opportunities to get to know one another. This way they are able to recognise when one member is not feeling up to scratch; be able to know that irritable or poor behaviour is an aberration and probably a sign that something is wrong, rather than a personality fault that will lead to less support just when he or she might need more. Meetings give people a chance too to air their feelings about aspects of care that have been painful for them (see Chapter 11) and this airing has been shown to improve both mental and physical health. If a team meeting is too difficult to convene, then regular one-to-one meetings will help to make young doctors feel necessary and belonging.
5 **Unskilled and unaware.** A series of studies has shown that most of us overestimate our skills. People who are particularly unskilled in certain areas are actually the most likely to overestimate their abilities. This seems to be a deficit in the capacity to distinguish accuracy from error, and it's been shown that, although it sounds like a paradox, improving their skills actually increases their capacity to recognise their limitations better. Where clinical work is concerned, in which uncertainty will continue to play a part throughout their careers, most medical students especially more likely to overestimate their skills. This growing area of individual differences around self-awareness of skill levels and tolerance of uncertainty is likely to have implications for doctors, particularly those working in some isolation where feedback may be less. In these days of error-reporting and learning from error, this may be particularly important to recognise, not only in terms of educational planning but also in the essential step of recognising that an error has been made at all. It does mean that an

initial lack of insight is normal rather than unusual, but the fact that accuracy of perception improves with increased skills is encouraging.

6 **Surveys.** Using an instrument like the 12-item GHQ over a whole organisation can give you an idea of where the most difficulties lie, though your absence and turnover figures will do that very well too. But surveys can also ask for more details on what is going wrong as well as suggestions for change. Once you find that you have an indication of high stress levels, a UK organisation has a duty of care under Health and Safety regulations, so needs to do what it can to relieve the problem; however, that is the whole point of the survey, so you would do that anyway. The more staff are involved and the more they can see that their concerns are noted and acted upon, the less stressed they will be. A diagonal slice of staff throughout the organisation – that is, across professions and down hierarchies – can provide a better view of what's happening than simply relying on middle management.

7 **Organisational factors.** As we outlined in Chapter 1, there are numerous job-related stressors within healthcare organisations, particularly now as they go through such violent changes around the world. One that needs addressing most urgently in terms of staff stress and patient safety are those to do with the increasing bed occupancy rates. Since it has been shown that this is related to the amount of anti-depressive medication used by doctors and nurses, and as various studies have shown that it also affects patient mortality, something has to change in the ways that increases in bed occupancy are managed. Other organisational ways to reduce or prevent stress include:
   - Thorough induction or orientation for new staff;
   - Consistency of staff within teams: this has been shown to improve patient safety but also offers better support to the team members;
   - Reliable administrative help;
   - Good performance management, including regular appraisal;
   - Regular voluntary multi-disciplinary groups to discuss harrowing or difficult events;
   - Hospital at Night so that those working still have the support of a team;
   - No clinical responsibilities after a night on call;
   - Regular social events;
   - Automatic counselling for anyone with a complaint against them or suspended.

8 **Modelling wellbeing and kindness.** If you are going to look after and reduce the stress levels of others, you need to show them how you look after yourself: having time for lunch, meeting socially, spending time talking to people (not just in corridors), talking about what worries you and what you are doing about it. Senior doctors always underestimate the

power they have over juniors and so just how much a little thing can affect them. Do spend time talking to your junior: it's quite frightening how little it's been shown to take for them to feel overwhelming grateful for a short chat about how it's going, and to report greater job satisfaction as a result!

9 **A board member for staff.** There is likely to be a board member with special responsibility for the quality of patient care. This person should also be responsible for the wellbeing of staff since the two are so intimately related. Having this addressed regularly at board level lets staff know that their health matters to the organisation, so regular communication about what is being discussed and addressed, need to take place. If your organisation is too small to have a board, then a member of the senior management team needs to take on this role.

13.2 Secondary interventions

When you are faced with a doctor whom you suspect has some sort of problem – whether they seem stressed or depressed, look like they have too many heavy nights, begun to make errors, or are badly behaved in the team or with patients – then it's important to intervene early. All doctors, whether senior or not, are prone to giving colleagues the benefit of the doubt till problems grow unavoidable, partly because of professional solidarity, of the anticipated stress of dealing with a disciplinary procedure, or because they think that 'there but for the grace of God go I', or they believe that confronting things might mean they lose an 'otherwise good doctor'. A list of behaviours compiled from workshops run by Professor Elisabeth Paice at London Deanery shows the main signs to look out for (Table 13.1).

In addition there are useful messages from management literature about the times when individuals' strengths can become overplayed, especially in times of stress. For example:

- Confidence and high self-esteem becomes arrogance and grandiosity,
- Conscientiousness becomes workaholic,
- Carefulness becomes obsessionality or over-caution,
- Charm becomes manipulation,
- Shrewdness becomes scepticism or cynicism.

It can be tricky to air your doubts, and they may possibly be unfounded, but once you've noticed something that doesn't feel right about a colleague, chances are there is a problem and facing it early is best. Reading the chapters on stress and depression (Chapters 5 and 6) and dealing with difficult people (Chapter 7) should help your decision-making. To make an interview easier, the list of questions opposite will give you a draft format for covering the possibilities of why the difficulties might be occurring. They allow you to be more accurate in

Table 13.1 Problematic working behaviours and examples

Behaviour	Examples
Rigidity	Difficulty recognising when corners must be cut Unwillingness to compromise Difficulty in prioritising Problems in dealing with ambiguity and uncertainty
Ward Rage	Flare-ups with colleagues Rows with nurses Inappropriate confrontations with patients Complaints and counter-complaints
The Disappearing Act	Arriving late, leaving early Excessive casual sick leave On-site but can't be found Bleep broken/lost Asking colleagues to hold bleep for an hour Not to be found in a crisis
The bypass syndrome	Patients ask to see a different doctor Nurses call senior colleagues first Junior colleagues go over the head, behind the back of the doctor Peers avoid being on duty with the doctor
Poor decision-making/poor judgment	Unsure whether to undertake a procedure Lack of confidence in own judgment/decisions Decisions made to avoid confrontations OR: Taking decisions others are better placed to take Decisions made with no clear line of reasoning Not knowing when to take advice/unwilling to seek advice Failure to recognise limitations/ask others for help Hasty judgments without considering all the facts

diagnosing the problem, but also provide less serious explanations which can often be missed, to the doctor's detriment. For example, the birth of a new baby, a partner's illness or job relocation are all life events which will result in a lack of sleep or worries and uncertainties for a period. Raising life events as a possible issue is likely to be a relief to the doctor, and the team can then rally round to give support which might otherwise have been absent (Table 13.2).

For questions 3–6 which cover illness and addiction, it is important that occupational health gets involved or, in organisations which do not have access to this, that referrals are made to appropriate specialists. For mental health problems and addiction there is often a specialised service for doctors provided locally, sometimes free, sometimes private. As a manager, it is worth

Table 13.2 A formula for exploring new difficulties

1. Is there a difficulty with clinical knowledge and skills? Might a deficiency in education, supervision or CPD be contributing to the problem?	This will take a skills assessment and educational input. It is possible for doctors to miss certain important aspects of education or to have had poor role models or supervision.
2. Have they had a recent life event?	Events such as separation, family illness, financial worries and even the birth of a child can affect both psychological and physical health temporarily.
3. Do they have a physical illness?	Is there a new or previously unknown physical illness? Has previous chronic illness worsened or relapsed? Could the behaviour be medication related?
4. Is the individual depressed or suffering from other mental illness?	Whether or not linked to life events, this can affect decision-making and memory and make an individual lose confidence and be irritable.
5. Might alcohol or substance misuse be involved?	The effects of alcohol are more obvious, but other drugs should be considered too.
6. Could there be a cognitive problem?	This may be caused by alcohol abuse, some chronic physical illness, a head injury (even one which seems mild) or by various dementias such as Alzheimer's disease.
7. Have work factors changed?	Are they losing sleep or working longer hours or with less support? Lack of sleep affects performance dramatically.
8. Are there team difficulties?	Has their principal team changed its function; is there new leadership or a new member who may have interpersonal problems with this doctor?
9. Have they recently been promoted?	It is possible they need support in learning leadership and management skills.
10. Have there been major organisational changes?	These may conflict with individual attitudes and values or may have changed their roles in some way.
11. Could issues relating to equality and diversity be a problem?	Consider factors that may disadvantage an individual from a minority group.
12. Is this really new behaviour or is it an exacerbation of longer-standing problems?	If problems are part of a pattern, the behaviour may result from a difficult personality or attitudes which are no longer acceptable.

finding out about these services and what they offer so that you can suggest them to the doctor with confidence. Psychotherapy or counselling will help with most cases of stress and depression, especially if treated early. And, as we outlined in Chapter 9 on addiction, this can be treated successfully, particularly in doctors, and there is no reason why he or she should not return to a successful career.

Questions 7–11 are organisational matters to be explored and hopefully rectified by your provision of team development, conflict resolution or various management courses for the doctor. In addition, it may be worth suggesting that they use a local counselling or coaching service, though it is important that they see that you are addressing the problem organisationally as well as offering the means of changing personally.

13.3 A long-standing problem

If, on investigation, the doctor has clearly shown these problems over time and in various organisations or departments, then you may want to have him or her assessed much more fully, especially if the problems remain after coaching or other appropriate remediation. In the United Kingdom, this could be done by the National Clinical Assessment Service, which assesses clinical, physical, mental and behavioural matters, but most disciplinary bodies also have the means to do this. Again, there is a real urge to get doctors back on track with their careers and sometimes a referral can be a life-saving act (see Chapter 9).

There are situations where senior doctors come up against a dilemma, as Robert's case describes.

> Robert is a partner in an inner city general practice, with a large proportion of Turkish patients. He has employed a locum GP for nine months now who speaks Turkish and is therefore invaluable to the practice. However, the locum has a number of potentially serious problems, both clinically and interpersonally. Robert felt he had to weigh up whether the added quality of care that this doctor provides in being able to accurately communicate with patients outweighs the potential clinical events that might damage patients. Robert raised his concerns at the regular meeting of the practice partners. He also got informal feedback from some of the senior non-medical staff at the practice. There was agreement that Robert's concerns were shared by others and that something needed to be done. Robert agreed to meet with the locum to talk things through. Unfortunately the response to gentle probing from Robert was not helpful – the locum GP denied that there were any problems. The practice then felt duty bound to gather evidence, which it passed on to the local Primary Care Trust.

And from time to time we are reminded that there are things which happen which are potentially even worse than possible incompetence. There have been a number of papers over the last few years concerning the 'rogue doctor' – ones who are involved in fraud, sexual relationships with patients, substance abuse and intentional harm to patients. It seems possible that some of these could have been spotted as early as medical school as studies which look back at the undergraduate years of doctors who are disciplined find that there were clear behavioural and psychological problems emerging even then. The prime concern of any doctor is patient safety and the quality of their care and so it is vitally important that doubts are dealt with when they appear. Again, work closely with human resources and senior management is important so that you know you are using the performance management system correctly from the start.

Gina is a Medical Director in a large teaching hospital. For some time she has been aware that one of her oncology colleagues has not been working as part of the team, has pushed his own ideas about chemotherapy regimes and most recently has tried to get the media behind his campaigns to utilise the latest non-agreed therapy options. This week he appeared on local television trying to get public support.

Gina called a meeting with him, which he thought was about her wanting to support his campaign. It was a difficult conversation, and left Gina no further forward. Next she decided to write to him formally to explain why his behaviour was unacceptable. His dismissive response to this made her realise the need for external help, so she sought the advice of the National Clinical Assessment Service. Their intervention included providing a framework explaining how this oncologist's behaviour fell outside professional boundaries. Challenged by this, the oncologist began to engage with Gina and, over time, his behaviour became more reasonable.

13.4 Getting help

Just because you're in a senior position now doesn't mean you are naturally going to know everything there is about management. Don't miss an opportunity to go on a relevant course nor to take time to understand yourself and how your style of management could be improved; 360 degree feedback is a good start in that it lets you become aware of how others see you. However, a good coach and mentor will let you take this forward and help you to change things you'd like to be different. And forming a good relationship with management is generally very worthwhile: most of them have even higher stress levels than you! And finally, don't be hard on yourself: it isn't an easy job but the more support you have around you, the better you'll do it.

Bibliography

Brewster JM, Kaufmann IM, Hutchison S, MacWilliam C. Characteristics and outcomes of doctors in a substance dependence monitoring programme in Canada: prospective descriptive study. *BMJ* 2008;**337**:a2098.

Cox J, et al. *Understanding Doctors' Performance.* 2005, Radcliffe Publishing, Abingdon.

Fahrenkopf AM, Sectish TC, Barger LK, et al. Rates of medication errors among depressed and burnt out residents: prospective cohort study. *BMJ* 2009;**336**:488–91.

Farmer JF, Return to work for junior doctors after ill-health. *Med J Aust* 2002;**177** (1 Suppl):S27–9.

Firth-Cozens J, Cording H, Ginsburg R. Can we select health professionals who provide safer care? *QSHC* 2003;**12**(Supp No.1):pi16–20.

Firth-Cozens J, King J. Are psychological factors linked to performance? In Cox J, et al. (eds) *Understanding Doctors' Performance.* 2005, Radcliffe Publishing, Oxford.

Ghodse H. *Addiction at Work: Tackling Drug Use and Misuse in the Workplace.* 2005, Gower Publishing Ltd, Eldershot England, Burlington USA.

Jones JW, Barge BN, Steffy BD et al, *Stress and medical malpractice: organisational risk assessment and intervention*, 1988; *J. Appl. Psychol*, 4, 727–35.

Landrigan CP, Rothschild JM, Cronin JW, et al. Effect of reducing interns' work hours on serious medical errors in intensive care units. *New Eng J Med* 2004;**351**:1838–48.

Leape L, Fromson JA. Problem doctors: Is there a system-level solution? *Ann Int Med* 2006;**144**:107–115.

McManus I, Winder B, Paice E. How consultants, hospitals, trusts and deaneries affect pre-registration house officer posts: a multilevel model. *Med Educ* 2002;**36**:35–44.

Nash S. *Turning Team Performance Inside Out: Team Types and Temperament for High-Impact Results.* 1999, Davies-Black Publishing, Palo Alto.

Papadakis MA, Hodgson CS, Teherani A, Kohatsu ND. Unprofessional behavior in medical school is associated with subsequent disciplinary action by a State Medical Board. *Acad Med* 2004;**79**:244–9.

Rafferty AM, Clarke SP, Cole J, et al. Outcomes of variation in hospital nurse staffing in England hospitals: cross-sectional analysis of survey data and discharge records. *Int J Nurs Stud* 2007;**44**:175–82.

Index